INFANT FEEDING 2000

A survey conducted on behalf of the Department of Health, the Scottish Executive, the National Assembly for Wales and the Department of Health, Social Services and Public Safety in Northern Ireland.

Becky Hamlyn, Sue Brooker, Karin Oleinikova, Sarah Wands

London: TSO

TSO

Published by TSO (The Stationery Office) and available from:

Online
www.tso.co.uk/bookshop

Mail, Telephone, Fax & E-mail
TSO
PO Box 29, Norwich, NR3 1GN
Telephone orders/General enquiries: 0870 600 5522
Fax orders: 0870 600 5533
E-mail: book.orders@tso.co.uk
Textphone 0870 240 3701

TSO Shops
123 Kingsway, London, WC2B 6PQ
020 7242 6393 Fax 020 7242 6394
68-69 Bull Street, Birmingham B4 6AD
0121 236 9696 Fax 0121 236 9699
9-21 Princess Street, Manchester M60 8AS
0161 834 7201 Fax 0161 833 0634
16 Arthur Street, Belfast BT1 4GD
028 9023 8451 Fax 028 9023 5401
18-19 High Street, Cardiff CF10 1PT
029 2039 5548 Fax 029 2038 4347
71 Lothian Road, Edinburgh EH3 9AZ
0870 606 5566 Fax 0870 606 5588

TSO Accredited Agents
(see Yellow Pages)

and through good booksellers

Published with the permission of the Department of Health on behalf of the Controller of
Her Majesty's Stationery Office.

First published 2002

ISBN 0113225709

Coventry University

Contents

Summary of main findings

The 2000 Infant Feeding Survey is the sixth national survey of infant feeding practices. The main aims of the survey are to provide national figures on the incidence, prevalence and duration of breastfeeding and other feeding practices adopted by mothers in the early weeks up to around nine months after the baby's birth.

Three stages of data collection were conducted and the survey is based on an initial national representative sample of nearly 9,500 mothers of babies born in the United Kingdom in 2000.

When comparing results with 1995, trend results should be seen in the context of changes in the population of mothers. Consistent with population changes, the sample of mothers in the 2000 survey were older and better educated when compared with the sample of mothers in 1995.

Incidence & duration of breastfeeding (Chapter 2)

Initial breastfeeding rates in 2000 were 71% in England and Wales, 63% in Scotland and 54% in Northern Ireland, this representing a significant rise since 1995 in all countries. The increase in breastfeeding incidence in England and Wales could be mainly accounted for by changes in the age and educational profiles of mothers. The increased incidences in Scotland and Northern Ireland, however, remained significant even after taking into account changes in the characteristics of the sample of mothers.

The highest incidences of breastfeeding were found among mothers from higher occupations, with the highest educational levels, aged 30 or over, from ethnic minority backgrounds, and among mothers of first (as opposed to later) babies.

Compared with 1995, significantly more mothers of later babies in 2000 were changing their feeding behaviour. In the United Kingdom, a quarter (26%) of mothers of later babies changed their behaviour by initiating breastfeeding, compared with less than a fifth (18%) in 1995.

Two-fifths (42%) of mothers were breastfeeding at six weeks, this halving to 21% of mothers breastfeeding at six months. Although the initial incidence of breastfeeding has increased significantly in all countries from 1995, only in Scotland did this increase remain significant beyond initiation at birth. Increases in prevalence of breastfeeding in Scotland were observed at all ages up to 9 months.

In the early weeks, breastfeeding mothers were more likely to be giving milk solely from the breast, as opposed to mixed milk feeds. Mothers from higher socio-economic groups and with a higher educational level were the most likely to provide milk from the breast alone at each stage of the survey.

The use of milk other than breast milk (Chapter 3)

In 2000, 30% of mothers in the United Kingdom did not breastfeed at all and gave infant formula as the sole source of nutrition from birth. By the first stage of the survey, when the babies were around four to ten weeks old, almost six in ten (58%) had switched entirely to infant formula milk, and three-quarters (75%) were using infant formula milk either entirely or in conjunction with breastmilk.

Among bottle-feeding mothers, two-thirds (64%) were giving a whey dominant as opposed to casein dominant formula at 4-10 weeks, this reducing to two-fifths (41%) at 4 – 5 months. By 8 – 9 months, a fifth (20%) of bottle feeding mothers were using whey dominant and three in ten (30%) casein dominant formula. Over a third (37%) were using follow-on formula milk at this stage, a significant increase from 25% in 1995.

At 8 – 9 months old, 8% had introduced cow's milk as the main milk drink (down from 15% in 1995). Just under three in ten (28%) had introduced it as a secondary drink and just under half (47%) were using it to mix food. In total, 54% had introduced cow's milk to their baby in some way by stage three of the survey (61% in 1995).

Antenatal care, smoking & drinking (Chapter 4)

Almost two-thirds (64%) of mothers of first babies had been to antenatal classes, a decline on the proportion in 1995 (70%).

Nine in ten mothers (92%) knew that increasing their intake of folic acid in early pregnancy could be beneficial, a significant increase from 1995 when 75% were aware of this. Almost nine in ten (89%) of all mothers had increased their intake in early pregnancy, mainly through supplementation (73%) rather than changing their diet (31%).

Just over a third (35%) of mothers in the United Kingdom smoked in the twelve months before or during their pregnancy. Three percent of mothers gave up smoking less than a year before pregnancy and were still not smoking at stage one of the survey and a further 11% gave up on confirmation of pregnancy and stayed quit. Thus a fifth (20%) of women in the UK continued to smoke throughout their pregnancy (although most cut down).

Six in ten mothers (61%) drank during pregnancy, a decline on the position in 1995, when two-thirds (66%) did so. The majority of those drinking in pregnancy (71%) drank less than one unit per week on average.

86% of smokers received information on the effect of smoking during pregnancy (no change from 1995). 77% of women who drank received advice on the effect of alcohol (up from 71% in 1995).

Choice of feeding method (Chapter 5)

Two-thirds (65%) of mothers in the United Kingdom said that they planned to breastfeed their baby, this figure ranging from 51% in Northern Ireland, to 60% in Scotland and 66% in England and Wales. There was a high correlation between intentions and behaviour.

First-time mothers were more likely to intend to breastfeed than mothers of later babies (70% compared to 60% in the UK). Among mothers of later babies, those who had breastfed their previous baby for at least 6 weeks were much more likely than mothers who had exclusively bottle fed their previous baby to plan to breastfeed (94% compared with 21%).

The most common reason for choosing to breastfeed was that breastfeeding was best for the baby's health, followed by convenience. The most common reason for choosing to bottle-feed was that it allowed others to feed the baby, followed by a dislike of the "idea" of breastfeeding.

Three-quarters (76%) of mothers were able to state a specific health benefit in breastfeeding. Knowledge about health benefits increased with age, educational level, and occupational level.

One in ten mothers who breastfed (9%) said that they felt pressured into this decision, rising to 12% of first-time mothers who breastfed. This pressure was mainly linked to midwives (76% of those feeling this way).

The birth & post-natal care (Chapter 6)

Mothers who experienced a delay before they first fed their baby were more likely to have given up breastfeeding in the first two weeks than were mothers who breastfed their baby immediately.

Use of formula milk in hospital was a strong indicator of mother giving up breastfeeding after leaving hospital. Two fifths (40%) of breastfeeding mothers whose babies had been given a bottle while in hospital had stopped breastfeeding within two weeks, compared with one in eight breastfeeding mothers (13%) whose babies had not been given a bottle.

32% of breastfeeding mothers experienced problems feeding their baby in hospital, and a similar proportion (35%) experienced feeding problems once they had left hospital. Mothers who did not receive help for these problems were more likely to have given up breastfeeding within the first two weeks than those who received help.

13% of bottle-feeding mothers experienced feeding problems in hospital and 12% experienced problems after they left. Compared with breastfeeding mothers who had problems, bottle-feeding mothers were more likely to cite difficulties relating to the health of the baby including vomiting and colic.

Feeding after the early weeks (Chapter 7)

One in six mothers (16%) had experienced problems feeding their baby between stages one and two, and one in eight (12%) between stages two and three. The problems experienced by bottle-feeding and breastfeeding mothers varied. Between the ages of about 4-10 weeks and 4-5 months, problems experienced by bottle-feeding mothers were mainly related to the baby (remaining unsatisfied after a feed, vomiting, illness or colic). Among breastfeeding mothers, however, problems tended to be centred on feeding techniques (baby refusing a bottle or painful breasts).

The majority of mothers (82% at stage two, 69% at stage three) reporting feeding problems had been given help or advice, most commonly received from the health visitor.

Reasons for giving up breastfeeding varied with the duration of breastfeeding. In the early weeks, baby rejecting the breast and painful nipples were the common reasons for cessation. In later weeks, up to about four months, mothers perceiving that they had insufficient milk was the most important factor. In later months, returning to work was the major reason for mothers reducing breastfeeding.

Mothers overall experience of breastfeeding was generally very positive. Nine in ten mothers (90%) who gave up breastfeeding within six weeks of birth would have liked to have breastfed for longer, and most mothers who breastfed (88%) said they would breastfeed another baby.

When the babies were around eight to nine months old, half (49%) of mothers were working, and in the majority of cases (68%) this was on a part-time basis. Mothers working part-time were more likely to continue breastfeeding while working, and 6% were still giving milk solely from the breast.

Additional drinks and supplementary vitamins (Chapter 8)

Just over half (55%) of mothers were giving their baby drinks other than milk at four to ten weeks. Mothers who where bottle feeding were more likely to have introduced other drinks (76%) than women who were breastfeeding (27%). Water was the most commonly mentioned additional drink at all three stages. Compared with 1995, there has been a marked shift away from sweetened drinks to unsweetened drinks and water.

At four to ten weeks, just 4% of babies received additional vitamins, 5% at four to five months and 10% at eight to nine months. These figures continue a longer-term trend in the declining use of this practice over the survey years.

A third (35%) of breastfeeding mothers were taking vitamin supplements and/ or iron tablets at stage one, falling to just over a quarter at the four and nine month stages (27% and 26% respectively).

Solid foods (Chapter 9)

Compared with 1995, mothers in 2000 were introducing solids later. By three months, a quarter of mothers (24%) had introduced solid foods, less than half the proportion recorded in 1995 (56%). The majority (85%) had introduced solids by the age of four months and by six months, virtually all babies had been introduced to solid food.

Despite this movement towards later introduction of solids, a high proportion of mothers was starting solid food earlier than thought desirable. Only half (49%) of mothers had introduced solids within the recommended window of four to six months (17 to 26 weeks), the large majority of the remainder introducing solids before 17 weeks (49% of all mothers).

Solid food tended to be introduced at a younger age among mothers in Northern Ireland, mothers of babies with heavier birth weights, those in lower occupational groups, and mothers with lower educational levels.

When babies were four to five months old, mothers giving solids were more likely to give commercially prepared babyfood (62%) than home-made food (38%), although by eight to nine months this had reversed, with seven in ten mothers (70%) giving home-made food compared with 52% giving babyfood.

In choosing which solid foods to give their baby, mothers at stage two most frequently took account of the nutritional value of foods, either in general terms or specifically relating to sugar, vitamins, gluten or salt. Half (47%) of stage three mothers avoided particular ingredients, most commonly sugar, salt and nuts. The most common reason for avoiding ingredients was allergies – this being a reason for a third (35%) of avoidances.

Acknowledgements

The authors would like to acknowledge and thank all those who contributed to making the survey such a success.

First and foremost, we would like to thank all the mothers who participated in the survey.

Their co-operation was essential to the success of the survey and ensured we achieved valuable insights into trends in infant feeding practices over recent years.

In the United Kingdom Health Departments, our thanks go to all who contributed. In particular, our thanks go to Dr. Sheela Reddy, Mrs Christine Carson and Mr John O'Shea for their support and assistance and to Mr. Robert Wenlock and Mr Anthony Boucher whose efforts were greatly appreciated in the preparation of the survey in its initial stages.

We would also like to thank the staff within the Birth Registration offices in England and Wales, Scotland and Northern Ireland and also the staff at ONS, Titchfield for the help and support they provided with the initial sampling of mothers. Thanks are also due to the staff in the Northern Ireland Statistics and Research Agency (NISRA) who co-ordinated the mailing and fieldwork operations in Northern Ireland.

Finally, we would like to thank all our colleagues at BMRB who have provided help and support in the organisation of questionnaire distribution, fieldwork and data analysis, especially our chief statistician, Mr Rick Loyd, and his colleague Andrew Parnell.

Notes to Tables

Base numbers are shown in italics and are weighted bases. Weighting factors have been adjusted so that the weighted sample size for all mothers is equal to the number of mothers responding at that stage. In previous survey years, weighting factors were adjusted to give the same total weighted sample size at each of the three stages of the survey, which will explain the differences in weighted sample sizes between years.

In general, very small bases have been avoided by combining adjacent categories. Where the base for a category is less than 50, the base and percentage are both shown in brackets [ ].

The **conventions** used in tables are as follows:

-        No cases

*   Percentage less than 0.5%

n/a   Data not available

[ ]   Percentage based on less than 50 cases

Percentages: Row or column percentages may add to 99% or 101% due to the effects of rounding

Statistical significance. Unless otherwise stated, changes and differences mentioned in the text are statistically significant at the 95% confidence level.

1

Introduction

1.1 Background & objectives

The 2000 Infant Feeding Survey is the sixth national survey of infant feeding practices. The survey was carried out by BMRB Social Research on behalf of the four United Kingdom Health Departments. Fieldwork in Northern Ireland was carried out by the Central Survey Unit of the Northern Ireland Statistics and Research Agency (NISRA).

Government policy has consistently supported breastfeeding as the best way of ensuring a healthy start for infants. In the 1970's, with the rates of breastfeeding declining, the COMA Working Party was set up to review infant feeding[1]. The recommendations included that mothers should be encouraged to breastfeed. It also recommended mothers to be discouraged from introducing solid foods to their infants before four months old. Subsequent reports about infant feeding have continued to endorse these recommendations[2,3,4].

The expert Working Party also recommended that a national survey be conducted to establish basic information about infant feeding practices. The first survey took place in 1975[5] and provided baseline statistics about infant feeding practices in England and Wales. Surveys have hence been conducted every five years since. The 1980[6] and 1985[7] surveys also covered Scotland, and from 1990[8] all four countries of the United Kingdom were covered by the infant feeding surveys. The 1975-1995 surveys were conducted by the Office of National Statistics.

The 1975 survey found that 51% of mothers in England and Wales breastfed at birth. In 1980, this proportion increased to 67%, and the figure for Scotland was 50%. The results of the 1985 survey showed that breastfeeding rates had not risen and, further, that there was a high rate of early discontinuation of breastfeeding.

Following the results of the 1985 Survey, the Department of Health engaged in a consultation process to find ways of promoting breastfeeding. This concluded in the setting up of the Joint Breastfeeding Initiative in 1988. The Initiative's aims were to encourage a closer working relationship between health professionals and voluntary organisations. In 1995, following the WHO/UNICEF adoption of the breastfeeding declaration, the National Breastfeeding Working Group was established. This was a multidisciplinary group whose objective was to publish a document, which is now known as, "*Breastfeeding – Good Practice Guidance to the NHS*"[9].

In 1995, the National Network of Breastfeeding Co-ordinators (NNBC) was established. The NNBC is a multidisciplinary group with representation from professional and voluntary organisations. The remit for this group is to build on the work of the National Breastfeeding Working Group in the promotion and protection of breastfeeding. This is done by stimulating and sustaining action at a local level and sharing ideas nationally, with the aim of increasing both the number of mothers who breastfeed and the length of time they continue to breastfeed.

The 1990 survey failed to show an improvement from 1985 in breastfeeding initiation rates for England & Wales and Scotland, although it was considered that the programmes of support described above had begun too recently to have had an impact on mothers' behaviour. (The 1990 survey also recorded a baseline breastfeeding initiation rate for Northern Ireland of 36%). The 1995 survey, however, did show an improvement in all countries of the United Kingdom.

The Infant Feeding Initiative was launched in 1999, as part of the Government's commitment to improve health inequalities. A budget of nearly £3m over a 3-year period from the Public Health Development Fund has enabled a range of activities to be undertaken. The aim of the initiative is to increase the incidence and duration of breastfeeding amongst those groups of the population where breastfeeding rates are lowest, as well as to help all women to make informed choices about how they feed their infant. Two National Infant Feeding Advisers have been appointed to support the work of the Infant Feeding Initiative

To date, 79 projects have been funded across all eight health regions in England to identify and communicate 'best practice' and to increase breastfeeding rates amongst those least likely to choose to breastfeed. A project has also been funded to find out whether midwives can be trained to make changes in their practice in relation, to a breastfeeding intervention and what impact a midwifery intervention would have to enable mothers to sustain their method of infant feeding.

Most recently, in July 2000, the *NHS Plan – A plan for investment and reform* was presented to Parliament which included a commitment by the Government for increased support for breastfeeding.

Given this background context, there is expected to be considerable interest in the results of the 2000 survey, in how trends in infant feeding have developed, and particularly among those subgroups of mothers where breastfeeding rates are lowest.

Smoking and drinking in pregnancy

The Infant Feeding Survey series has also been used to track the proportion of mothers who smoke and drink during pregnancy, and to look at patterns of smoking and drinking behaviour before, during and after the birth.

Of particular relevance to the 2000 survey, the Tobacco White Paper '*Smoking Kills*' was published in December 1998 and contains the Government's anti-smoking strategy. This White Paper highlighted smoking among pregnant women as a key area, and included the target:

> 'To reduce the percentage of women who smoke during pregnancy from 23% to 15% by the year 2010; with a fall to 18% by the year 2005'

The 2000 survey therefore measures progress towards this target[10].

Aims of the survey

The main aims of the 2000 survey match those of the earlier Infant Feeding Surveys and are as follows:

- To establish how infants born in 2000 are being fed and to provide national figures on the incidence, prevalence and duration of breastfeeding.
- To examine trends in infant feeding practices over recent years, in particular since 1995.
- To investigate the factors associated with mothers' feeding intentions and with the feeding practices adopted in the early weeks.
- To establish the age at which solid foods are introduced and to examine weaning practices up to nine months.

As in 1995, the survey involved approaching a sample of mothers when their babies were aged four to ten weeks (Stage 1), with follow-up questionnaires at four to five months (Stage 2) and at about nine months (Stage 3).

1.2 Definitions used in the survey

A number of terms defined for the infant feeding surveys since 1975 are used in this report. The definitions are as follows.

Breastfed initially refers to all babies whose mothers put them to the breast, even if this was on one occasion only.

Incidence of breastfeeding refers to the proportion of sampled babies who were breastfed initially.

Prevalence of breastfeeding refers to the proportion of all sampled babies who were wholly or partially breastfed at specified ages.

Duration of breastfeeding is the length of time for which breastfeeding continued at all, regardless of when non-breast milk and other drinks or foods were introduced.

Mothers giving milk only from the breast refers to babies who were being provided with milk solely from the breast, with no additional formula or cows' milk. However, these babies may also have been receiving solids and/or additional non-milk drinks.

Stages of the survey

The approximate age of babies at the different stages of the survey were as follows:

Stage 1: babies aged 4-10 weeks
Stage 2: babies aged 4 to 5 months
Stage 3: babies aged 8 to 9 months

1.3   Summary of survey methodology

Full details of survey methodology have been provided in Appendix I. However, a summary is provided below.

- A total of 13,112 births were selected from all births occurring in the period August 19th-October 19th 2000: 7382 in England & Wales, 3113 in Scotland and 2617 in Northern Ireland. In England and Wales, the babies selected were clustered within 100 registration sub-districts. In Scotland and Northern Ireland, births were sampled across all registration districts.

- In selecting the samples, births to mothers whose partner was classified from his birth registration details as social class V, where no father was recorded, or where the social class details were unclassified, were given twice the chance of selection as mothers whose partner was classified to social classes I-IV.

- The initial despatch of questionnaires was conducted during October-December 2000, with the aim of contacting mothers when their babies were about six weeks old. Three reminders were sent to all mothers who had not responded to the previous mailouts. The overall response rate at Stage 1 was 72% (n=9492).

- For the second stage of the survey, a further despatch took place in January/February 2001 to all mothers who responded at Stage 1. Two postal reminders were sent, followed by an interviewer visit to all mothers who had not responded to the postal reminders. The response rate at Stage 2, based on all responding at Stage 1, was 87% (n= 8299).

- For the third stage of the survey, a despatch took place during June/July 2001 to all mothers who responded at Stage 2. As in Stage 2, this was followed by two postal reminders and an interviewer visit. The response rate at Stage 3, based on all those responding at Stage 2, was 88% (n=7267).

- At Stage 1, the data were weighted to correct for differential sampling of mothers with different social classes, from different countries, and to correct for non-response bias by social class group. Further weighting was applied at Stages 2 and 3 to correct for further non-response bias introduced through sample attrition at the later stages.

1.4   Making comparisons with results from the 1995 survey

One of the main aims of the 2000 survey is to provide data on trends in infant feeding, so this section considers the main factors which might affect comparisons over time.

There are four factors which should be taken into consideration.

Sampling error

The results of sample surveys are subject to sampling error due to the chance variations between a particular sample and the whole population from which it has been drawn. When comparing results from two separate samples, each will be subject to sampling error and so observed changes over time may be attributable to sampling variation. Sampling errors are affected both by the size of the sample subgroup on which the estimates are based and by the variability of the particular measure within the sample. They will also be affected by the complexity of the sample design. Further details and examples of standard errors for key variables are given in Appendix III.

Non-response

Both surveys are subject to possible biases due to non-response. The 2000 survey was shown to have differential response rates by social class group at all stages, and the data were weighted to correct for this (see Appendix I). The achieved samples in each year, after weighting, can be validated by comparison with registration data for all births in the relevant year (see Appendix II). The comparison shows that the 2000 weighted sample was similar, in terms of the characteristics compared, including mothers' age and social class, to all births in the United Kingdom.

Changes in the characteristics of mothers

Any significant changes in the characteristics of the sample of mothers in different years will affect the interpretation of trend data, and this will be particularly influential if these characteristics are themselves associated with key survey measures. Comparison of the main characteristics of mothers in the 1995 and 2000 samples are shown in Tables 1.1 to 1.4 and further details are given in Appendix II (Tables II.4 to II.11). In line with changes in the population as a whole, the 2000 survey showed clear differences from the 1995 sample on key measures. Many of these changes continue trends which were also evident between 1990 and 1995.

- Mothers in the 2000 survey were older than those sampled in 1995, in each of the countries of the United Kingdom. In England and Wales, 46% of women were aged 30 or over compared with 40% in 1995 (*Table 1.1*). Tables II.5 and II.6. in Appendix II show that this increase is concentrated within the higher social class and more educated subgroups of the sample.
- Mothers in 2000 were more educated than mothers in the 1995 sample. In England and Wales, 28% of mothers were educated to higher education age (19 or over) compared with 20% in 1995. (*Table 1.2*)
- The 2000 survey showed a reduction in the proportion of mothers coded to social class "unclassified/no partner" which makes the distributions of social class difficult to compare. However, there is no evidence to suggest that the social class distribution has changed. (*Table 1.3*)
- Babies in 2000 were slightly more likely than babies in 1995 to be born as a first baby rather than a second or subsequent baby. In England and Wales, 47% of babies were first babies, compared with 45% in 1995. (*Table 1.4*)

Table 1.1
Distribution of sample by mother's age and country (1995 & 2000)

	England & Wales		Scotland		Northern Ireland	
	1995 %	2000 %	1995 %	2000 %	1995 %	2000 %
Under 20	6	7	6	6	5	6
20-24	19	18	18	16	16	15
25-29	34	28	34	29	35	30
30-34	28	30	30	31	29	33
35+	12	16	12	18	14	16
All aged 30+	40	46	41	49	43	49
Base: All mothers	4598	5441	1863	2274	1476	1779

Table 1.2
Distribution of sample by age at which mother completed full-time education and country (1995 & 2000)

	England & Wales		Scotland		Northern Ireland	
	1995 %	**2000** %	**1995** %	**2000** %	**1995** %	**2000** %
16 or under	45	37	44	36	32	25
17 or 18	35	34	33	33	43	40
19 or over	20	28	23	31	24	34
Base: All mothers	*4598*	*5441*	*1863*	*2274*	*1476*	*1779*

Table 1.3
Distribution of sample by social class as defined by current or last occupation of husband or partner by country (1995 & 2000)

	England & Wales		Scotland		Northern Ireland	
	1995 %	**2000** %	**1995** %	**2000** %	**1995** %	**2000** %
I	7	7	8	7	6	5
II	25	25	21	24	22	21
IIINM	8	9	7	9	11	10
All non-manual	39	41	36	41	38	36
IIIM	24	26	24	26	22	29
IV	11	11	12	11	8	11
V	4	4	4	5	4	3
All manual	38	40	39	42	38	43
Unclassified/no partner	22	19	25	18	24	21
Base: All mothers	*4598*	*5441*	*1863*	*2274*	*1476*	*1779*

Table 1.4
Distribution of sample by birth order and country (1995 & 2000)

	England & Wales		Scotland		Northern Ireland	
	1995 %	**2000** %	**1995** %	**2000** %	**1995** %	**2000** %
First baby	45	47	47	49	39	41
Later baby	55	53	53	51	61	59
Base: All mothers	*4598*	*5441*	*1863*	*2274*	*1476*	*1779*

Age of babies at the three survey stages

Many of the questions on the survey relate to feeding practices at the time the mother completes the questionnaire. Thus, comparison of these variables over time may also be affected by differences in the age distribution of the babies at each stage of the survey. This of course does not affect variables which are based on specific ages of the baby such as duration of breastfeeding, age of introduction of solid foods etc. However, it may affect comparison of questions which were based on the mother's behaviour and opinions at the time she completed the questionnaire e.g. whether the baby has had a developmental check up by the time the mother completed the Stage 1 questionnaire, or whether the baby was receiving additional drinks at the time of the Stage 2 survey. Differences can result from changes in sampling registration procedures, or simply because of changes in the speed with which mothers respond to the postal request. There were two main changes between 1995 and 2000 which have influenced the age profile of babies.

- Firstly, there was a change in the method of sampling births for England, Wales and Scotland by ONS. In 2000, the mailout was staggered over eight phases, which meant that mothers received questionnaires earlier than they would have done in 1995, when the mailout was less staggered. As a result of this, at Stage 1, babies in the England & Wales and Scotland sample were, on average, younger than those in the 1995 sample (46 days compared with 57 days in England and Wales, and 54 days compared with 71 days in Scotland). In Northern Ireland, where mailout procedures remained similar, there was no change in the average age of babies. As a result of the changes in England and Wales and Scotland, fewer babies in 2000 were aged between six and ten weeks (in the UK 54% compared with 78% in 1995). In 2000, 84% of babies were found to be aged between four and ten weeks. Therefore, in this report, the age of the babies at Stage 1 of the survey has been described as "*four to ten weeks*" rather than "*six to ten weeks*" as in previous surveys.
- Secondly, there was a difference in the pattern of response from mothers at Stages 2 and 3 in 2000 (see Appendix I). In 2000, a lower rate of mothers than in 1995 responded to the postal enquiry, and a higher rate of mothers responded to the interviewer enquiry. Thus, although the overall response rates at Stages 2 and 3 were similar for the two survey years, the 2000 survey picked up more mothers in the later stages of fieldwork. As a result of this, the difference between the ages of babies between 1995 and 2000 at Stage 1 began to even out by Stage 3. At Stage 1, in the UK, babies were on average 10 days younger in 2000 than in 1995. By Stage 2, this gap had widened to around 2 weeks. However, by Stage 3, babies in 2000 had the same average age as babies in 1995. See *Table 1.5*.

Table 1.5
Age of baby at the three stages of the survey

	England & Wales		Scotland		Northern Ireland		United Kingdom	
	1995 %	2000 %	1995 %	2000 %	1995 %	2000 %	1995 %	2000 %
Mean age of babies at:								
Stage 1 (days)	57 days	46 days	71 days	54 days	61 days	60 days	58 days	48 days
Stage 2 (nearest week)	22 wks	20 wks	23 wks	21 wks	24 wks	20 wks	22 wks	20 wks
Stage 3 (nearest week)	39 wks	39 wks	41 wks	41 wks	39 wks	39 wks	39 wks	39 wks
Percentage of babies								
Aged 6-10 weeks at Stage 1	78	50	76	80	86	82	78	54
Aged 4-10 weeks at Stage 1	n/a	86	n/a	88	n/a	83	n/a	84
Base:	*4598*	*5441*	*1867*	*2274*	*1476*	*1778*	*5181*	*9492*

1.5 Further notes about comparisons between data from 1995 and 2000

Comparison of survey universes

In the infant feeding surveys between 1980 and 1990 inclusive, data were collected from England & Wales and Scotland only. Thus, historically, data on the total sample have been presented on Great Britain. This practice was continued to a large extent in the 1995 report when making comparisons with previous surveys. However, in 2000, data for the total sample have been exclusively presented on the United Kingdom. Thus, when a table shows longer-term trends, it is sometimes the case that data pre-2000 are presented on Great Britain, with 2000 data presented on the United Kingdom. As the data from Northern Ireland contributed relatively little to the overall totals, due to the effects of weighting, the differences between Great Britain and the United Kingdom are negligible in the large majority of cases. Nevertheless, where trend tables show data from different years based on different universes, this has been clearly noted in the table.

Comparison of weighted bases

In both 1995 and 2000, weighted bases are shown in all tables. In 1995, the bases used in tables were scaled to a single base, regardless of which stage the data related to. Thus when data were analysed on "all mothers" this was uniformly set to 5018, whether the data originated from Stage 1, 2 or 3. In 2000, however, a decision was made to scale the weighted base to the total number of responding mothers at each stage, as this gives readers a much better indication of the actual number of respondents included in the base. Thus "all mothers" varies from 9492 at Stage 1, to 8299 at Stage 2, to 7267 at Stage 3. Therefore, when making comparisons between the survey years, the large differences in weighted bases can be attributed to changes in the scaling of bases rather than changes in numbers of responding mothers.

As in 1995, when results for each country are shown separately, they are weighted only to compensate for differential non-response and the over-sampling of lower social class groups. When results are based on the United Kingdom as a whole, then the additional weighting to compensate for over-sampling in Scotland and Northern Ireland is also applied.

1.6 Analysis by socio-economic classifications

In all past infant feeding surveys up to and including 1995, mothers socio-economic position was defined by social class based on current or most recent occupation of their husband or partner. However, in the 2000 survey there have been two important changes in the method of classifying mothers according to their socio-economic position.

- The first major change has been in the system of classification. In 2001, following the Census, the system of classifying respondents for government surveys in terms of their socio-economic position changed. Formerly, and in all previous infant feeding surveys, occupations were classified according to Social Class. However, this survey changes to the new ONS classification - the **National Statistics Socio-Economic Classification (NS-SEC)**[11]. The new classification aims to differentiate positions in terms of their "employment relations" rather than "skill" level. Occupations are no longer classified according to the "manual/non-manual" divide.
- Secondly, a decision was made to base the classification in 2000 on **mother's** as opposed to **partner's** occupation. Previous surveys have retained the practice of using the partner's occupation to classify mothers, which has had the advantage of maintaining comparability throughout the survey series. However, this practice is no longer considered desirable. In particular, in this survey where we are looking at the opinions and behaviours of mothers, it is likely that their **own** socio-economic position could influence their behaviour. Thus, the classification is based on mother's occupation at the time of the first stage of the 2000 survey (including any job from which they were taking maternity absence). Where a mother was not working at the time of the Stage 1 survey, the classification has been based on the mother's previous occupation. Mothers who had never worked are classified separately. Mothers whose classification was not coded due to missing or insufficient information provided in the questionnaires (10% of all mothers) are also identified separately.

Analyses based on social class

Although the 2000 data have been analysed by the new mother's NS-SEC throughout this report, where it has been of interest to look at changes within socio-economic groupings over time, we have presented the data on social class of partner as in previous years. As in 1995, the analyses in this report use information taken from the survey questionnaires about the husband's or partner's occupation to assign social class. However, where information given in the questionnaire was insufficient to code social class, then social class based on information collected at registration was used as a proxy. A social class could not be assigned to mothers who were neither married nor living with a partner, nor where incomplete information was given about the partner's occupation. Data for these two groups are shown separately in the tables.

Analyses based on mother's NS-SEC

The distribution of the 2000 sample by NS-SEC is shown in Table 1.6, for the full eight-class categorisation and the aggregated five-class and three-class versions of the scale. A decision was made to use the simplified three-class categorisation (higher, intermediate, and lower occupations) together with "never worked" as this provided the most balanced scale.

Table 1.6
Distribution of 2000 sample by mother's NS-SEC for the eight, five and three-class versions

8 classes	%	5 classes	%	3 classes	%
Large employers & higher managerial occupations	3	Managerial & professional occupations	29	Higher occupations	29
Higher professional occupations	3				
Lower managerial and professional occupations	23				
Intermediate occupations	17	Intermediate occupations	17	Intermediate occupations	20
Small employers and own-account workers	3	Small employers and own-account workers	3		
Lower supervisory and technical occupations	6	Lower supervisory and technical occupations	6	Lower occupations	28
Semi-routine occupations	14	Semi-routine & routine occupations	22		
Routine occupations	8				
Never worked and long-term unemployed	14	Never worked and long-term unemployed	14	Never worked and long-term unemployed	14
Unclassified	10	Unclassified	10	Unclassified	10
Base: *All Stage 1 mothers*	*9492*		*9492*		*9492*

It is of interest to look at the relationship between the new NS-SEC and the old partner's social class, in order to investigate how well the two scales correlate. Of course, a very high degree of correspondence should not necessarily be expected as NS-SEC was based on the mother's current or previous occupation whereas social class was based on the partner's occupation details. Nevertheless Table 1.7 shows that there is a reasonably high level of correspondence between the two scales. A half (53%) of mothers classified to higher occupations would have been classified as social class I or II under partner's class and two-thirds (64%) would have been classified to any non-manual social class. The large majority of the remainder (21%) would have been placed in the highest of the manual categories, IIIM.

Mothers classified to intermediate occupations were more evenly split between non-manual (49%) and manual (41%) occupations under the social class categorisation. Mothers classified to lower occupations would predominantly have been placed in either a manual social class (54%) or as no partner/unclassified (23%), this latter category including father's who had never worked. Mother who had never worked would disproportionately have been classified as either having no partner or partner unclassified (43%) or in manual occupations (40%).

Mothers who gave insufficient information to code their NS-SEC were more likely than average to have been classed under the social class schema as having no partner or partner unclassified (29% compared with 19% of all mothers). They were correspondingly somewhat less likely to be classified in a non-manual social class group (32% compared with 40% overall). Thus this suggests that more of the mothers whose NS-SEC was unclassified in fact should have been classified to lower occupations or never worked, given the high correspondence between manual and unclassified social classes and those at the lower end of the NS-SEC scale, as discussed above. Therefore, it should be noted that it is possible that the NS-SEC scale may be slightly skewed in favour of higher rather than lower occupations.

Table 1.7
Distribution of partner's social class based on current or former occupation of husband or partner by mother's socio-economic classification (NS-SEC) (United Kingdom, 2000)

	Mother's NS-SEC					
	Higher occupations	Intermed-iate occu-pations	Lower occupat-ions	Never occupat-ions	Unclass-ified	All mothers
I & II	53	37	17	12	26	32
IIINM	11	12	6	5	6	9
All non-manual	**64**	**49**	**23**	**17**	**32**	**40**
IIIM	21	28	34	21	23	26
IV & V	8	13	21	19	16	15
All manual	**29**	**41**	**54**	**40**	**39**	**41**
No partner/unclassified	8	11	23	43	29	19
Base (all Stage 1 mothers)	*2790*	*1905*	*2618*	*1277*	*902*	*9492*

[1] Department of Health and Social Security *Present day practice in infant feeding* Report on Health and Social Subjects 9. HMSO (London:1974)

[2] Department of Health and Social Security. *Present day practice in infant feeding: 1980.* Report on Health and Social Subjects 20. HMSO (London: 1980)

[3] Department of Health and Social Security. *Present day practice in infant feeding: third report.* Report on Health and Social Subjects 32. HMSO (London: 1988)

[4] Department of Health. *Weaning and the weaning diet. Report of the working group on the Weaning Diet of the committee on Medical Aspects of Food Policy* Report on Health and Social Subjects 45. HMSO (London: 1994)

[5] Martin J. *Infant Feeding 1975: attitudes and practice in England and Wales.* HMSO (London: 1978)

[6] Martin J and Monk J *Infant Feeding 1980.*OPCS (London: 1982)

[7] Martin J and White A *Infant Feeding 1985.*OPCS (London: 1988)

[8] White A, Freeth S and O'Brien M *Infant feeding 1990.* HMSO)London: 1992)

[9] *Breastfeeding Good Practice Guide to the NHS* DH1995

[10] See section I.4 in Appendix I for a note on changes to smoking questions between 1995 and 2000.

[11] See www.statistics.gov.uk/methods_quality/ns-sec/default.asp

2

Incidence & duration of breastfeeding

Summary

Initial incidence of breastfeeding

- Initial breastfeeding rates in 2000 were 71% in England and Wales, 63% in Scotland and 54% in Northern Ireland. In all countries, there was a significant increase in breastfeeding incidence between 1995 and 2000.

- The increase in breastfeeding incidence in England and Wales since 1995 could be mainly accounted for by changes in the age and educational profiles of mothers. The increased incidences in Scotland and Northern Ireland, however, remained significant even after taking into account changes in the characteristics of the sample of mothers.

- The highest incidences of breastfeeding were found among mothers from higher occupational groups, with the highest educational levels, aged 30 or over, from ethnic minority backgrounds, among mothers of first (as opposed to later) babies, and mothers with previous experience of breastfeeding.

- The increase in breastfeeding incidence between 1995 and 2000 was concentrated within mothers at the lower end of the social class scale, within the manual subgroup, mothers with no partner, and partners' occupations unclassified.

Changes in feeding behaviour between previous and subsequent babies

- Compared with 1995, significantly more mothers of later babies in 2000 were *changing* their feeding behaviour. In the United Kingdom, a quarter (26%) of mothers of later babies changed their behaviour by initiating breastfeeding, compared with less than a fifth (18%) in 1995.

- Those mothers who had changed their behaviour from bottle to breast feeding between children were younger, less well-educated and from a lower socio-economic grouping when compared with mothers who had breastfed at both occasions.

Prevalence & duration of breastfeeding

- Although the initial incidence of breastfeeding has increased significantly in all countries from 1995, only in Scotland did this increase extend beyond birth. Increases in prevalence of breastfeeding in Scotland were observed at all ages up to 9 months.

- In 2000, among those women who did breastfeed initially, the proportion still breastfeeding at 6 weeks remained similar in England & Wales and Scotland compared to 1995. However, in Northern Ireland there was a sharper decline in the rates of breastfeeding over the first few weeks compared with 1995.

- Scottish women who breastfeed do so for the longest with 40% still breastfeeding at six months, compared with 34% in England & Wales and 21% in Northern Ireland.

Mixed milk feeding

- In the early weeks, breastfeeding mothers were more likely to be giving milk solely from the breast than to give mixed breastmilk and formula feeds. Mothers from higher socio-economic groups and with a higher educational level were the most likely to provide milk from the breast alone at each stage of the survey. Mothers of black and Asian ethnic origin showed a preference for mixed over sole breastfeeding at each stage of the survey, in contrast to white mothers.

This chapter presents the key statistics about initiation of breastfeeding, the length of time women continue to breastfeed, how women change their feeding behaviour between previous and subsequent babies, as well as the prevalence of breastfeeding and mixed milk feeding. Variations by different demographic subgroups are explored.

2.1 Incidence of breastfeeding

Incidence of breastfeeding is defined as the **proportion of babies who were breastfed initially**. This includes all babies who were put to the breast at all, even if this was on one occasion only.

2.1.1 Longer-term trends

Table 2.1 and Figure 2.1 illustrate the trends in the incidence of breastfeeding by country for all available years since 1980. The historical data shows that between 1985 and 1990, initiation rates in England & Wales and Scotland remained broadly stable, followed by a significant increase between 1990 and 1995. This trend has continued over the period between 1995 and 2000. Breastfeeding incidence in England and Wales now stands at 71%, an increase of 3 percentage points since 1995, and 7 percentage points since 1990. A marked increase can be observed in Scotland, where rates have risen to 63% from 55% in 1995, and from 50% in 1990. Breastfeeding incidence in Northern Ireland (54%) continues to be lower than elsewhere in the United Kingdom, although this too represents a very significant rise since 1995 (45%), which in turn was higher than in 1990 (36%).

Table 2.1, Figure 2.1

Table 2.1
Incidence of breastfeeding by country (1980, 1985, 1990, 1995 and 2000)

	England & Wales					Scotland					Northern Ireland			United Kingdom		
	1980	1985	1990	1995	2000	1980	1985	1990	1995	2000	1990	1995	2000	1990	1995	2000
Percentage who breastfed initially	67	65	64	68	71	50	48	50	55	63	36	45	54	62	66	69
Base (all Stage 1 mothers)	3755	4671	4942	4598	5441	1718	1895	1981	1863	2274	1497	1476	1778	5533	5181	9492

Figure 2.1
Incidence of breastfeeding by country: 1980 to 2000
Base: All Stage 1 mothers

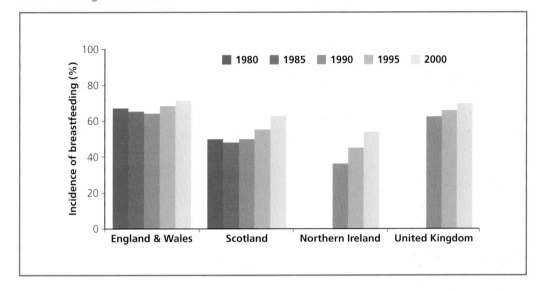

Although these changes represent a significant increase in breastfeeding in each country, it is important to place the results in the context of changes in the composition of the sample since 1995. As detailed in section 1.4, there have been some important shifts in the profile of new mothers since 1995. The 2000 sample contained greater proportions of mothers aged 30 or over, and mothers who had continued in education beyond the age of 19, these changes continuing trends evident since 1985[1]. Both of these factors are strongly associated with the incidence of breastfeeding (see section 2.1.2). Moreover the groups which have increased in size are those with higher breastfeeding rates. Explanation of observed national trends in breastfeeding is therefore complicated by the fact that, even if the rates for different groups had remained constant, overall rates would have increased simply as a result of changes in the composition of the sample.

The technique of **standardisation** was used to separate the contribution of compositional change from what might be termed "real" change over the period since 1985. The calculated standardised rates show the breastfeeding rates which would have been expected in 1990, 1995 and 2000 if the samples of mothers in those two surveys had had the same characteristics as the 1985 sample (1990 in the case of Northern Ireland).

Analysis was carried out to standardise for the combined effects of age and educational level within each country.

As already seen in Table 2.1, survey estimates of the incidence of breastfeeding in England and Wales were 64% in 1990, 68% in 1995 and 71% in 2000. The standardised rates, assuming that the distributions of age and education of the sample had remained the same as in 1985 were 62% in all three years. Thus the observed change in breastfeeding between 1995 and 2000 could be attributed to changes in the sample composition.

Changes in sample composition also had some effect on estimates of incidence in Scotland, but the standardised rates still indicate a fairly substantial increase in the incidence of breastfeeding between 1995 and 2000 (from 48% to 54%). This follows a much smaller increase between 1990 and 1995 (from 46% to 48%).

In Northern Ireland, a similar pattern was evident, standardisation removing some but not all of the observed increase in breastfeeding between 1995 and 2000. Even after standardisation, the estimated incidence of breastfeeding rose from 41% to 47%.

Table 2.2

Table 2.2
Estimated incidence of breastfeeding standardised by composition of the sample, by country

	1985	1990	1995	2000
	Percentage who breastfed initially			
England & Wales				
Unstandardised percentage	65	64	68	71
Standardised for mother's age and age finished full-time education	65	62	62	62
Scotland				
Unstandardised percentage	48	50	55	63
Standardised for mother's age and age finished full-time education	48	46	48	54
Northern Ireland				
Unstandardised percentage	n/a	36	45	54
Standardised for mother's age and age finished full-time education	n/a	36	41	47

2.1.2 Variations in the incidence of breastfeeding

Birth order

Previous surveys have shown that the incidence of breastfeeding is higher among mothers of first rather than later babies. This continued to be the case in 2000 and was seen in all countries. Across the United Kingdom, three-quarters (74%) of first-time mothers breastfed their babies initially compared with two-thirds (65%) of mothers of subsequent babies. It is interesting to note that across the time period between 1995 and 2000, breastfeeding rates have increased by a greater degree among second or later babies as compared with first-time babies, which has led to a reduction in the gap between the breastfeeding behaviour of first and later mothers. This is explored further in section 2.2.

Table 2.3, Figure 2.2

Socio-economic status of mothers

In all past infant feeding surveys up to and including 1995, mothers' socio-economic position was defined by social class based on current or most recent occupation of their husband or partner. However, as described in section 1.6, since 1995 there have been two important changes in the method of classifying mothers according to their socio-economic position. The first major change has been to base the classification on **mother's** as opposed to **partner's** occupation. The second major change has been to change the system of classification to the new Office of National Statistics (ONS) classification - the **National Statistics Socio-Economic Classification (NS-SEC),** which was introduced in 2001. Full details of the new socio-economic classification and given in Section 1.6, together with a discussion of the implications of using the new scale in terms of its relationship to partner's social class.

The following section gives a detailed breakdown of breastfeeding incidence by mothers' NS-SEC. However, in order to examine any change in the incidence of breastfeeding within socio-economic groups over time, we have also provided some comparative data based on partner's social class.

Table 2.3
Incidence of breastfeeding by birth order and country (1995 and 2000)
Base: All Stage 1 mothers

	England & Wales		Scotland		Northern Ireland		United Kingdom	
	1995	2000	1995	2000	1995	2000	1995	2000
			Percentage who breastfed initially					
First birth	74	75	61	67	52	59	72	74
Second or later birth	62	66	50	59	40	51	60	65
Bases (Stage 1 mothers)								
First birth	*2076*	*2560*	*867*	*1115*	*578*	*729*	*2355*	*4448*
Second or later birth	*2522*	*2881*	*996*	*1159*	*898*	*1049*	*2845*	*5044*

Figure 2.2
Incidence of breastfeeding by birth order and country: 1995 and 2000

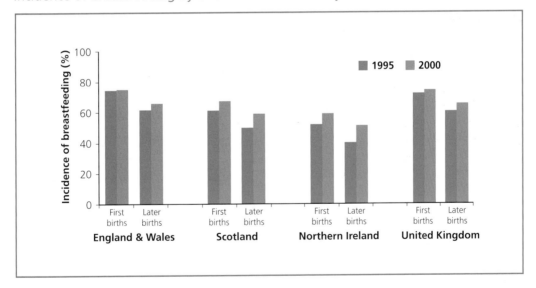

Mother's socio-economic classification (NS-SEC)

Although the analysis is now based on a different classification system, a similar trend to that seen in previous surveys can be observed, whereby mothers classified into higher occupations were more likely to initiate breastfeeding than their counterparts in lower occupations. In the United Kingdom, 85% of mothers classified to higher occupations breastfed initially, compared with 73% of mothers in intermediate and 59% in lower occupations. The lowest initiation rate was seen among those mothers who had never worked, this figure being 52%.

Compared with England and Wales, breastfeeding initiation rates were lower in Scotland and Northern Ireland for each of the socio-economic groups, reflecting the general trend seen in Table 2.1.

Table 2.4, Figure 2.3

Table 2.4
Incidence of breastfeeding by mother's socio-economic classification (NS-SEC) and country, 2000

	England & Wales	Scotland	Northern Ireland	United Kingdom
	Percentage who breastfed initially			
Higher occupations	86	80	76	85
Intermediate occupations	75	64	56	73
Lower occupations	60	53	45	59
Never worked	54	41	33	52
Unclassified	68	62	48	66
All babies	**71**	**63**	**54**	**69**
Bases (Stage 1)				
Higher occupations	*1600*	*702*	*484*	*2791*
Intermediate occupations	*1090*	*461*	*363*	*1906*
Lower occupations	*1499*	*624*	*503*	*2619*
Never worked	*740*	*268*	*232*	*1277*
Unclassified	*510*	*218*	*196*	*901*
All babies	***5441***	***2274***	***1778***	***9492***

Figure 2.3
Incidence of breastfeeding by mother's socio-economic classification (NS-SEC) and country: United Kingdom 2000
Base: All Stage 1 mothers

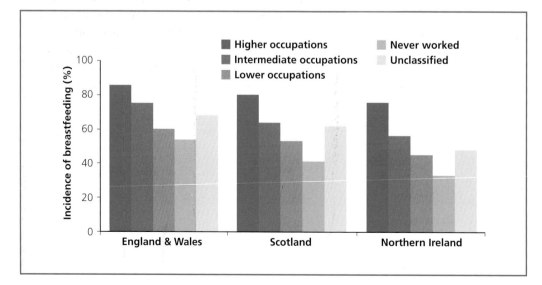

Social class (as defined by the current occupation of the husband or partner)

This section provides an analysis of data by social class in order to examine any changes in the breastfeeding incidence within social class categories over time. The analyses in this report use information taken from the survey questionnaires about the husband's or partner's occupation to assign social class. However, where information given in the questionnaire was insufficient to code social class, then social class based on information collected at registration was used as a proxy. A social class could not be assigned to mothers who were neither married nor living with a partner, nor where incomplete information was given about the partner's occupation. Data for these two groups are shown separately in the tables.

Trend data for the individual countries are shown in Table 2.5. In England and Wales, a significant increase was observed between 1995 and 2000 in social class group IIINM. In Scotland, significant increases were observed in non-manual social class groups I and II, manual group IV, and no partner. In Northern Ireland, significant increases were found in II, IIINM, IIIM and IV.

Figure 2.4 displays the change in incidence between survey years for the United Kingdom as a whole. In the United Kingdom, significant increases over time were observed towards the lower end of the social class scale in IIINM, in the aggregate manual category, and in the no partner/unclassified subgroups.

Table 2.5, Figure 2.4

Age at which mother completed full-time education

As in previous years, mothers in 2000 who left full-time education at 16 years old were least likely to breastfeed, while those who had continued in education beyond 18 years were most likely to do so. The association between breastfeeding and the mother's educational level was evident in all countries. For example, in England and Wales, nine in ten mothers leaving school after 18 breastfed compared to just over half of mothers who left school at 16.

Looking at trend data, it can be seen that there have been no significant changes in the breastfeeding rates according to educational level within England or Wales, or overall at the UK level. However, within Scotland and Northern Ireland, increases are evident in the two lower educational level categories (although only significant in the 16 or under category). This indicates that the overall rise in breastfeeding rates between 1995 and 2000 in these two countries was concentrated among the less well-educated sectors of the population.

Table 2.6

Table 2.5
Incidence of breastfeeding by social class based on current or last occupation of husband or partner, by country (1995 & 2000)*

	England & Wales		Scotland		Northern Ireland		United Kingdom	
	1995	2000	1995	2000	1995	2000	1995	2000
	Percentage who breastfed initially							
I	91	91	82	90	79	87	90	91
II	82	84	71	79	59	68	81	83
IIINM	72	79	65	65	55	66	71	77
All non-manual	**82**	**84**	**72**	**78**	**61**	**70**	**80**	**83**
IIIM	65	65	52	58	41	52	63	64
IV	58	62	48	58	38	51	57	61
V	50	59	56	47	36	38	50	57
All manual	**61**	**64**	**51**	**56**	**40**	**51**	**60**	**63**
Unclassified	62	71	56	65	33	[47]	61	70
No partner	49	53	30	41	24	33	46	51
All births	**68**	**71**	**55**	**63**	**45**	**54**	**66**	**69**
Bases (Stage 1)								
I	*303*	*369*	*149*	*162*	*83*	*96*	*346*	*639*
II	*1150*	*1373*	*398*	*552*	*318*	*370*	*1275*	*2366*
IIINM	*354*	*465*	*138*	*206*	*156*	*179*	*402*	*823*
All non-manual	*1807*	*2207*	*685*	*920*	*557*	*645*	*2023*	*3828*
IIIM	*1113*	*1398*	*439*	*597*	*383*	*519*	*1254*	*2461*
IV	*483*	*579*	*220*	*247*	*121*	*186*	*546*	*1010*
V	*164*	*218*	*65*	*112*	*56*	*55*	*185*	*382*
All manual	*1760*	*2195*	*724*	*957*	*560*	*760*	*1985*	*3853*
Unclassified	*294*	*167*	*105*	*54*	*107*	*[25]*	*330*	*279*
No partner	*737*	*871*	*347*	*343*	*251*	*348*	*843*	*1532*
All births	*4598*	*5441*	*1863*	*2274*	*1476*	*1778*	*5181*	*9492*

* The percentages in 2000 have changed slightly since the first release of data. This is due to changes in the derivation of social class data between publication of the first release and the main report, whereby mothers whose social class was originally recorded as "unclassified" were later reclassified using the registration data as a proxy where available.

Mother's age

As in previous years, there was a strong association between breastfeeding and mother's age across all survey countries. In Scotland, for example, breastfeeding rates ranged from three in ten among mothers aged under 20 to seven in ten among mothers aged 30 or over. When looking at trend data, significant rises can be seen across all except the youngest age group within Scotland, and within the 25-29 and 30+ age-groups in Northern Ireland.

Table 2.7

Figure 2.4
Incidence of breastfeeding by social class based on current or last occupation of husband or partner (United Kingdom, 1995 & 2000)

Base: All Stage 1 mothers

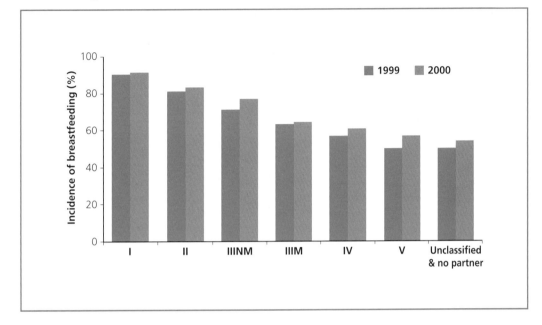

Table 2.6
Incidence of breastfeeding by age completed full-time education, by country (1995 & 2000)

	England & Wales		Scotland		Northern Ireland		United Kingdom	
	1995	2000	1995	2000	1995	2000	1995	2000
	Percentage who breastfed initially							
16 or under	53	55	39	46	26	38	51	54
17 or 18	74	72	59	63	46	50	72	70
Over 18	90	89	80	83	68	71	88	88
All births*	**68**	**71**	**55**	**63**	**45**	**54**	**66**	**69**
Bases (Stage 1)								
16 or under	*2042*	*2009*	*805*	*813*	*471*	*446*	*2275*	*3436*
17 or 18	*1600*	*1875*	*618*	*743*	*634*	*716*	*1810*	*3289*
Over 18	*913*	*1507*	*432*	*708*	*356*	*603*	*1049*	*2683*
All births*	***4598***	***5441***	***1863***	***2274***	***1476***	***1778***	***5181***	***9492***

* Includes some cases where mother's education was not known

Table 2.7
Incidence of breastfeeding by mother's age & country (1995 & 2000)

	England & Wales		Scotland		Northern Ireland		United Kingdom	
	1995	2000	1995	2000	1995	2000	1995	2000
	Percentage who breastfed initially							
Under 20	46	49	24	31	24	24	43	46
20-24	57	60	43	53	34	41	55	58
25-29	68	69	55	63	46	54	66	67
30 or over	76	79	65	70	50	62	74	78
All births*	**68**	**71**	**55**	**63**	**45**	**54**	**66**	**69**
Bases (Stage 1)								
Under 20	*284*	*383*	*121*	*143*	*73*	*103*	*319*	*557*
20-24	*883*	*973*	*342*	*360*	*240*	*269*	*986*	*1670*
25-29	*1566*	*1544*	*629*	*655*	*521*	*526*	*1765*	*2703*
30 or over	*1855*	*2520*	*771*	*1112*	*640*	*873*	*2100*	*4428*
All births*	***4598***	***5441***	***1867***	***2274***	***1476***	***1778***	***5181***	***9492***

* Includes some cases where mother's age was not known

Ethnicity

There were clear cultural differences between the breastfeeding rates of mothers from different ethnic backgrounds. Mothers from ethnic minority groups (Asian, Black, mixed and other ethnic origin) were considerably more likely to breastfeed at birth compared with white mothers. Two in three white mothers breastfed at birth, compared with around eight to nine in ten of each of the ethnic minority groups.

Comparative data on ethnicity from 1995 was not available.

Table 2.8, Figure 2.5

Table 2.8
Incidence of breastfeeding by ethnicity (United Kingdom, 2000)

	%	Base
White	67	*8608*
Asian	87	*275*
Black	95	*185*
Mixed	86	*93*
Other	86	*66*
All Stage 1 births*	**66**	***9492***

* Includes some cases where ethnicity was not known

Figure 2.5
Incidence of breastfeeding by ethnicity: United Kingdom, 2000
Base: All Stage 1 mothers

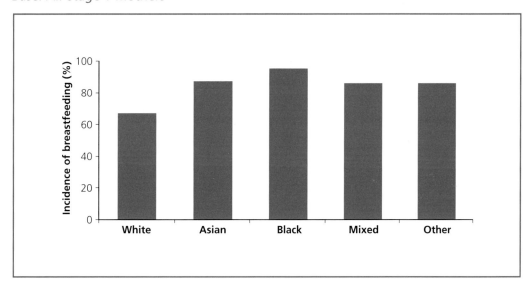

Region

As in 1995, there was a regional differential in the incidence of breastfeeding mothers, with the highest rates found in the south - London & the South East, and the South West & Wales – and the lowest rates found in the North, together with Scotland and Northern Ireland. Rates varied from a low of 54% in Northern Ireland to a high of 81% in London and the South East. By year, increases can be observed across all regions with the exception of the Midlands and East Anglia.

Table 2.9

Table 2.9
Incidence of breastfeeding by region (United Kingdom 1995 & 2000)

	1995	2000	Base 1995	Base 2000
	%	%	%	%
London & South East	76	81	1818	1884
South West & Wales	70	74	684	821
Midlands & East Anglia	64	65	907	1029
North	56	61	1190	1684
Scotland	55	63	1867	2274
Northern Ireland	45	54	1476	1778
All Stage 1 births*	**66**	**69**	*5181*	*9492*

* Includes some cases where region was not known

2.2   **Changes in feeding behaviour between previous and subsequent babies**

In Table 2.3 it was shown that the incidence of breastfeeding was higher among mothers of first rather than later babies. Moreover, there has been clear evidence from previous surveys that the likelihood of a mother breastfeeding a second or subsequent baby is strongly correlated to her experience of feeding previous children. This has led to the targeting of feeding information and advice to first-time mothers.

This pattern is again repeated in 2000. Overall, across the United Kingdom, 65% of babies of all later births were breastfed at least initially. Among mothers who had not breastfed their previous child, this proportion was 26%, rising to 68% of mothers breastfeeding previous children for less than six weeks and 96% of mothers breastfeeding previous children for at least six weeks. Similar patterns are evident within all countries.

Although this trend echoes a similar one found in 1995, there have been some important shifts within the general trend. In 1995, less than a fifth (18%) of mothers who solely bottle fed their previous child changed to breastfeeding for their subsequent child. In 2000, as noted above, over a quarter (26%) of this group changed their behaviour from bottle to breastfeeding, and a similar differential can be observed within each country (from 15% to 22% in Scotland, and from 12% to 20% in Northern Ireland). This is a key finding as it indicates that, compared with five years ago, more women are *changing* their feeding behaviour between children from bottle to breast.

There has also been a positive shift in the proportion of mothers choosing to breastfeed who had breastfeed their previous child, but for less than six weeks. In 1995, in Scotland and Northern Ireland, less than half of mothers in this subgroup breastfed their subsequent child. This situation may have arisen if, for example, a mother had difficulties breastfeeding her previous child leading her to abort this feeding practice at an early stage, this then deterring her from attempting to breastfeed the next time.

However, in 2000, there has been a marked shift within these two countries in the proportion of mothers who stopped at an early stage with their previous child but have attempted to breastfeed again with their later child. Nearly two-thirds (63%) of these mothers in Scotland opted to breastfeed again, a rise of 17 percentage points since 1995, and in Northern Ireland, three-quarters of this subgroup of mothers chose to breastfeed again, a steep rise of 31 percentage points.

These figures indicate that messages about the benefits of breastfeeding are getting through to all mothers, not simply first-time mothers, and those who have had successful breastfeeding experiences in the past.

Following this theme, it is interesting to look at the duration of breastfeeding among mothers who did not breastfeed their previous baby, and whether mothers who did breastfeed their previous child are now breastfeeding longer. This is explored in section 2.4.2

Table 2.10, Figure 2.6

Table 2.10
Incidence of breastfeeding among mothers of more than one child according to length of time for which previous children were breastfed, by country (1995 and 2000)

	England & Wales		Scotland		Northern Ireland		United Kingdom	
	1995	2000	1995	2000	1995	2000	1995	2000
	Percentage who breastfed initially							
Never breastfed	18	27	15	22	12	20	18	26
Breastfed for less than 6 weeks	60	68	46	63	43	74	59	68
Breastfed for 6 weeks or more	93	96	93	95	88	93	93	96
All later births*	**62**	**66**	**51**	**59**	**40**	**51**	**60**	**65**
Bases (Stage 1 mothers)								
Never breastfed	*782*	*987*	*414*	*453*	*462*	*526*	*926*	*1793*
Breastfed for less than 6 weeks	*525*	*556*	*184*	*207*	*156*	*194*	*584*	*966*
Breastfed for 6 weeks or more	*1154*	*1210*	*374*	*462*	*262*	*289*	*1267*	*2068*
All later births*	***2522***	***2881***	***996***	***1159***	***898***	***1049***	***2845***	***5044***

* Includes some cases where mother's method of feeding previous children was not known

Figure 2.6
Incidence of breastfeeding by experience of feeding previous child and country: 1995 to 2000

Base: All later births

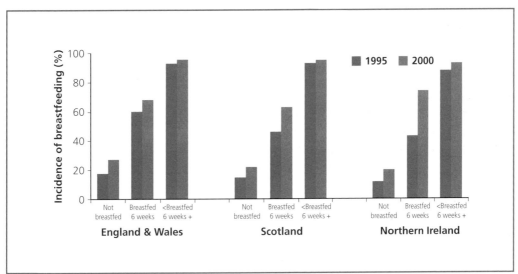

Given that there has been such a significant shift in the proportion of women who chose to breastfeed their current baby, even if they didn't breastfeed their previous child or only breastfed them for a relatively short period, it is interesting to look at the profile of these subgroups of mothers in more detail.

Table 2.11 displays the profile of women in each of three categories according to mother's age, age left full-time education, and socio-economic classification (NS-SEC). The three categories are:

i. Did not breastfeed previous baby, breastfed current baby ("Bottle to breast")
ii. Breastfed previous baby for less than 6 weeks, breastfed current baby ("repeat breastfeeders")
iii. Breastfed previous baby for 6 weeks or more, breastfed current baby ("repeat long-term breastfeeders")

Table 2.11

Table 2.11
Characteristics of mothers according to whether they changed their feeding behaviour between previous and current babies (United Kingdom, 2000)

	Bottle to breast	Repeat breastfeeders	Repeat long-term breastfeeders
	%	%	%
Mother's age			
Under 25	18	12	8
25-29	31	26	20
30+	51	61	71
Age completed FT education			
16 or under	48	37	24
17-18	36	40	33
19+	15	23	42
Mother's NS-SEC			
Higher occupations	20	28	41
Intermediate occupations	17	25	23
Lower occupations	32	30	19
Never worked	21	9	9
Unclassified	10	8	8
*Base (Stage 1 mothers with previous children breastfeeding initially)**	*468*	*659*	*1987*

* Some figures are calculated on bases slightly lower than these depending on level of missing data

The table shows that there are strong demographic differences between those who have changed their feeding behaviour between babies from bottle to breast, and those who are "repeat long-term breastfeeders". Compared with mothers who had breastfed their baby on both occasions, those who had changed their feeding behaviour from bottle to breast were disproportionately younger, less well-educated and from lower occupational groups. For example, 18% of "bottle to breast" mothers were aged under 25, 48% left education at age 16 or under and 53% were classified as either lower occupations or never worked. The equivalent figures for "repeat long-term breastfeeders" are 8%, 24% and 28%. The characteristics for those we have defined as "repeat breastfeeders" occupy a middle position between the two.

Thus the figures show that the shift from bottle to breast between babies was concentrated among those mothers in the more socially excluded groups of the population.

2.3   Prevalence of breastfeeding

Prevalence of breastfeeding is defined as the **proportion of all babies who are being breastfed at specific ages, even if they are also receiving infant formula or solid food**.

2.3.2   Trend data by country

Table 2.12 illustrates the changes in the prevalence of breastfeeding by country since 1995. As already seen, the initial rates of breastfeeding – at birth – are higher in 2000 than in 1995 for all countries. However, in England & Wales and Northern Ireland this improvement does not continue when looking at later ages. In England & Wales there was no improvement in breastfeeding rates at any age beyond birth, and in Northern Ireland there were small, but non-significant, improvements at later ages. Thus, although more women were now breastfeeding at birth, there was still a high fall-out in the early weeks. In England and Wales, the prevalence of breastfeeding drops from 71% to 43% by six weeks, and in Northern Ireland the corresponding figures are 54% and 26%.

However, in Scotland, where we have already seen an 8 percentage point increase in breastfeeding rates at birth, this improvement continues at all ages up eight months. At one week, a half of all mothers are still breastfeeding (an improvement of 4 percentage points on 1995), and by four months three in ten are still breastfeeding (an improvement of 6 percentage points). Compared with the other countries, mothers in Northern Ireland were much less likely to breastfeed at all ages.

Table 2.12

2.3.3   Variations in the prevalence of breastfeeding

Birth order

As shown in Table 2.2 earlier, mothers of first babies were more likely to initiate breastfeeding at birth. However, when looking at prevalence in the later weeks, the figures begin to even out, indicating that there is a higher fall-out rate among first-time mothers compared with mothers of second or subsequent babies. For example, by six weeks, breastfeeding prevalence stands at 42% for both first and later babies which means that 32% of first-time mothers stopped breastfeeding within the first 6 weeks compared with 23% of mothers of later babies.

Table 2.13

Table 2.12
Prevalence of breastfeeding at ages up to 9 months by country (1995 and 2000)

Age of baby	England & Wales		Scotland		Northern Ireland		United Kingdom	
	1995	2000	1995	2000	1995	2000	1995	2000
	Percentage breastfeeding at each age							
Birth	68	71	55	63	45	54	66	69
1 week	58	57	46	50	35	37	56	55
2 weeks	54	54	44	47	32	34	53	52
6 weeks	44	43	36	40	25	26	42	42
4 months (17 weeks)	28	29	24	30	12	14	27	28
6 months (26 weeks)	22	22	19	24	8	10	21	21
8 months (35 weeks)*	16	17	14	18	6	7	15	16
9 months (39 weeks)*	14	14	13	15	5	7	14	13
Base (all babies at Stage 3)	*4598*	*4112*	*1863*	*1718*	*1476*	*1437*	*5181*	*7267*

* Based on a reduced number of cases excluding those babies who had not reached this age by Stage 3

Table 2.13
Prevalence of breastfeeding at ages up to 9 months by birth order (United Kingdom, 2000)

	First birth	Later birth	All babies
	Percentage breastfeeding at each age		
Birth	74	65	69
1 week	58	54	55
2 weeks	54	51	52
6 weeks	42	42	42
4 months (17 weeks)	27	29	28
6 months (26 weeks)	19	23	21
8 months (35 weeks)*	14	18	16
9 months (39 weeks)*	11	15	13
Base (all babies at Stage 3)	*3367*	*3900*	*7267*

* Based on a reduced number of cases excluding those babies who had not reached this age by Stage 3

Mother's socio-economic classification

Table 2.14 shows that the differential observed between the different socio-economic groups at birth (Table 2.4) continues at all ages beyond birth. For example, 60% of women in higher occupations were breastfeeding at six weeks compared with 28% of women in lower occupations and 26% of those who had never worked.

Table 2.14

Table 2.14
Prevalence of breastfeeding at ages up to 9 months by mother's socio-economic classification (NS-SEC) (United Kingdom, 2000)

	Higher occupations	Intermed-iate occu-pations	Lower occupat-ions	Never occupat-ions	Unclass ified	All mothers
	Percentage breastfeeding at each age					
Birth	85	73	59	52	65	69
1 week	73	58	42	36	52	55
2 weeks	69	55	38	34	50	52
6 weeks	60	42	28	26	41	42
4 months (17 weeks)	43	27	17	17	26	28
6 months (26 weeks)	31	21	13	13	21	21
8 months (35 weeks)*	22	17	10	11	18	16
9 months (39 weeks)*	18	15	8	9	15	13
Base (all babies at Stage 3)	*2314*	*1558*	*1982*	*769*	*643*	*7267*

* Based on a reduced number of cases excluding those babies who had not reached this age by Stage 3

Age at which mother completed full-time education

We have already seen that mothers who continued their education beyond the age of 18 are more likely to breastfeed their babies at birth compared with those who completed their education sooner (Table 2.6). Table 2.15 below shows that this differential breastfeeding prevalence continued at all later ages. For example, two-thirds (64%) of mothers in the highest educational category were breastfeeding at six weeks compared with around a quarter (27%) of mothers in the lowest educational category.

Table 2.15

Ethnic group

Table 2.8 illustrated that mothers from ethnic minority backgrounds were more likely to breastfeed at birth compared with white mothers. The data on prevalence of breastfeeding at various ages shows more detailed differences between the ethnic groups. Asian mothers were more likely than white mothers to be breastfeeding at all ages up until four months, at which point the figures begin to become more balanced between the two groups. However, Black mothers were more likely than white mothers to breastfeed at all ages up to and including nine months. Those with "other" and "mixed" ethnic backgrounds were the most committed in terms of breastfeeding, with nearly half (46%) breastfeeding at six months and three in ten (31%) breastfeeding at nine months.

Table 2.16

Table 2.15

Prevalence of breastfeeding at ages up to 9 months by age left full-time education (United Kingdom, 2000)

	16 or under	17 or 18	Over 18	All babies**
	Percentage breastfeeding at each age			
Birth	54	69	87	69
1 week	40	54	75	55
2 weeks	37	51	72	52
6 weeks	27	40	64	42
4 months (17 weeks)	16	25	48	28
6 months (26 weeks)	11	18	37	21
8 months (35 weeks)*	9	13	28	16
9 months (39 weeks)*	7	11	24	13
Base (all babies at Stage 3)	2510	2595	2104	7267

* Based on a reduced number of cases excluding those babies who had not reached this age by Stage 3
**Base includes some cases where mother's education was not known

Table 2.16

Prevalence of breastfeeding at ages up to 9 months by mother's ethnic group (United Kingdom, 2000)

	White	Asian	Black	Mixed & other**	All mothers
	Percentage breastfeeding at each age				
Birth	67	87	95	86	69
1 week	54	72	77	73	55
2 weeks	51	66	77	72	52
6 weeks	41	51	69	65	42
4 months (17 weeks)	28	28	46	50	28
6 months (26 weeks)	21	23	31	46	21
8 months (35 weeks)*	15	19	26	41	16
9 months (39 weeks)*	13	17	19	31	13
Base (all babies at Stage 3)	6761	148	104	106	7267

* Based on a reduced number of cases excluding those babies who had not reached this age by Stage 3
** Categories combined due to low base sizes

2.4   Duration of breastfeeding

The duration of breastfeeding refers to the **length of time that mothers who breastfed initially continue to breastfeed even if they were also giving their baby other milk and solid foods.**

The results presented in this section relate only to mothers who ever breastfed and show the proportion who were still breastfeeding at one week, two weeks, six weeks, four months, six months and nine months.

2.4.1   Trend data by country

Table 2. 17 compares the duration of breastfeeding in 1995 and 2000 by country. The rates in England and Wales and Scotland were similar between 1995 and 2000 for all ages up to six weeks. However, there was a statistically significant increase in the proportion of breastfeeding mothers in England & Wales who were still doing so at four months; 45% of mothers who breastfed initially were still doing so at four months, compared with 42% in 1995. Similarly, in Scotland, the proportion of women still breastfeeding at four months increased from 45% to 50%, and a significant rise is also observed at six months (from 35% to 40%). When comparing the results in Scotland against those in England and Wales, it can be seen that, among those who breastfeed initially, Scottish women breastfed for longer on average than women in England and Wales. By six months, 40% of Scottish women were still breastfeeding compared to 34% of women in England and Wales.

As in 1995, Northern Ireland showed a steeper decline than other countries in the proportion who continued to breastfeed at later ages, with a particularly sharp fall after one week. Nearly three in ten women (28%) who attempt breastfeeding at birth give up within the first week. This compares with only 15% and 17% in England & Wales and Scotland respectively. In fact, contrary to other trends which tend to show an improvement in breastfeeding rates between 1995 and 2000, there has been a significant fall in the proportion of women in Northern Ireland still breastfeeding in the early weeks, from 79% to 72% at one week, and from 73% to 66% at two weeks. Thus although a greater proportion of women in Northern Ireland were attempting to breastfeed in 2000 compared with 1995, the duration is now shorter.

By six weeks, half (51%) of women who initially started to breastfeed in Northern Ireland were still breastfeeding, compared with around two-thirds in the other countries. By nine months, the rate drops to one in nine breastfeeding mothers (11%), compared with 19% in England & Wales and 23% in Scotland.

Table 2.17, Figure 2.7

Table 2.17
Duration of breastfeeding for those who were breastfed initially by country (1995 and 2000)

Age of baby	England & Wales		Scotland		Northern Ireland		United Kingdom	
	1995	2000	1995	2000	1995	2000	1995	2000
				Percentage still breastfeeding				
Birth	100	100	100	100	100	100	100	100
1 week	86	85	84	83	79	72	85	84
2 weeks	81	80	79	78	73	66	80	79
6 weeks	65	65	66	67	56	51	65	64
4 months (17 weeks)	42	45	45	50	27	30	42	44
6 months (26 weeks)	32	34	35	40	19	21	32	34
9 months (39 weeks)*	21	19	24	23	11	11	21	19
Base (all Stage 3 mothers breastfeeding initially)	*3106*	*2900*	*1029*	*1082*	*659*	*778*	*3410*	*4760*

* Based on a reduced number of cases excluding those babies who had not reached this age by Stage 3

Figure 2.7
Duration of breastfeeding for those who were breastfed initially by country : United Kingdom, 2000

Base: All Stage 3 mothers breastfeeding initially

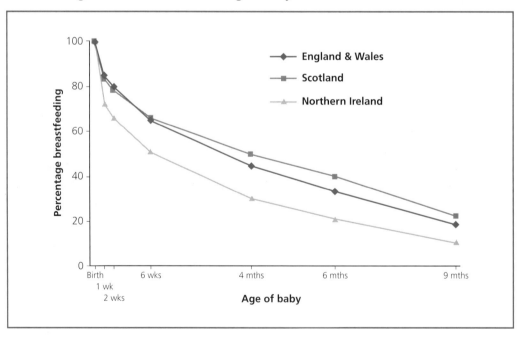

2.4.2 Variations in the duration of breastfeeding

Birth order & previous experience of breastfeeding

As found in previous surveys, mothers of second or later babies breastfeed for longer than mothers of first babies. Data for the United Kingdom in Table 2.18 show that 69% of later babies were still breastfed at six weeks compared with 60% of first babies. By six months the figures drop to 39% of later, compared to 29% of first, babies.

Table 2.18

Table 2.18
Duration of breastfeeding for those who were breastfed initially by birth order
(United Kingdom, 2000)

	First birth	Later birth	All babies
	Percentage still breastfeeding		
Birth	100	100	100
1 week	82	86	84
2 weeks	77	82	79
6 weeks	60	69	64
4 months (17 weeks)	40	49	44
6 months (26 weeks)	29	39	34
9 months (39 weeks)*	15	23	19
Base (all Stage 3 mothers breastfeeding initially)	*2486*	*2537*	*5023*

* Based on a reduced number of cases excluding those babies who had not reached this age by Stage 3

Section 2.2 showed that that a relatively high proportion (26%) of mothers who bottle fed their previous child switched to breastfeeding for their subsequent child. However, when we look at the duration of breastfeeding by mothers' experience of breastfeeding previous children, there are some clear differences between the subgroups. Table 2.19 shows that, for the subgroup of women who chose to breastfeed after exclusively bottle feeding their previous child, there was a sharp decline in breastfeeding over the first six weeks. Over a third (37%) gave up within the first week, and by six months only one in six of these mothers (16%) were still breastfeeding.

Among those mothers who breastfed their previous child, the duration of breastfeeding subsequent children was longer, although this varied depending on how long they breastfed their previous child. Among those mothers who breastfed their previous child for less than six weeks, there was a still a relatively high fall-out in the early weeks with one in three (30%) giving up in the first week; and two-thirds of mothers who breastfed their earlier child for less than six weeks ceased breastfeeding within the same timeframe for their later child.

However, those mothers who breastfed their child for at least six weeks previously, continued to breastfeed their later child for significantly longer. Nearly nine in ten (86%) were still breastfeeding at six weeks, and half of these mothers continued to breastfeed for at least six months.

Table 2.19, Figure 2.8

Table 2.19

Duration of breastfeeding for those who were breastfed initially by mother's previous experience of breastfeeding (United Kingdom, 2000)

	Previous child not breastfed	Breastfed previous child < 6 weeks	Breastfed previous child 6 weeks +	All second & later
	Percentage still breastfeeding			
Birth	100	100	100	100
1 week	63	70	96	86
2 weeks	56	60	94	82
6 weeks	38	35	86	69
4 months (17 weeks)	22	17	65	49
6 months (26 weeks)	16	12	52	39
9 months (39 weeks)*	12	5	34	23
Base (Stage 3 mothers breast-feeding initially with previous children)	*335*	*479*	*1598*	*2537*

* Based on a reduced of cases excluding those babies who had not reached this age by Stage 3

** Includes some cases where previous experience of breastfeeding not known

Figure 2.8

Duration of breastfeeding for those who were breastfed initially by previous experience of breastfeeding : United Kingdom, 2000

Base: All Stage 3 mothers breastfeeding initially with previous children

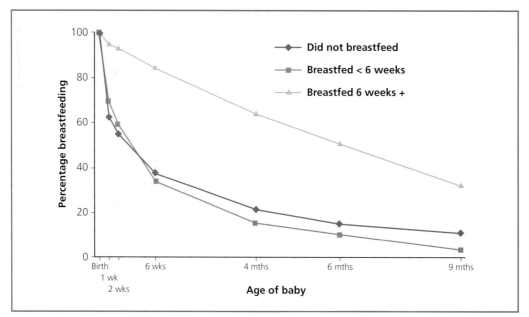

Mother's socio-economic classification

There is a strong relation between the duration of breastfeeding and mother's socio-economic status, with a longer duration of breastfeeding in mothers from higher occupational groups. In 2000, three-quarters (75%) of women who breastfed initially and were classified to higher occupations were still doing so at six weeks compared with about half (53%) of women in lower occupations. By six months, the equivalent figures are 41% and 27%.

Breastfeeding mothers who had never worked continued breastfeeding for longer on average than mothers in the lowest occupational group. Three-fifths (60%) were still breastfeeding at 6 weeks, and a third (34%) continued until at least six months.

Table 2.20, Figure 2.9

Table 2.20
Duration of breastfeeding for those who were breastfed initially by mother's socio-economic classification (NS-SEC) (United Kingdom, 2000)

	Higher occupations	Intermed-iate occu-pations	Lower occupat-ions	Never occupat-ions	Unclass-ified	All mothers
	Percentage still breastfeeding					
Birth	100	100	100	100	100	100
1 week	90	83	77	82	85	84
2 weeks	86	78	71	77	81	79
6 weeks	75	60	53	60	67	64
4 months (17 weeks)	55	40	34	42	45	44
6 months (26 weeks)	41	32	27	34	36	34
9 months (39 weeks)*	24	22	18	24	26	19
Base (all Stage 3 mothers breastfeeding initially)	*1964*	*1130*	*1136*	*378*	*415*	*5023*

* Based on a reduced number of cases excluding those babies who had not reached this age by Stage 3

Figure 2.9
Duration of breastfeeding for those who were breastfed initially by mother's socio-economic classification : United Kingdom, 2000

Base: All Stage 3 mothers breastfeeding initially

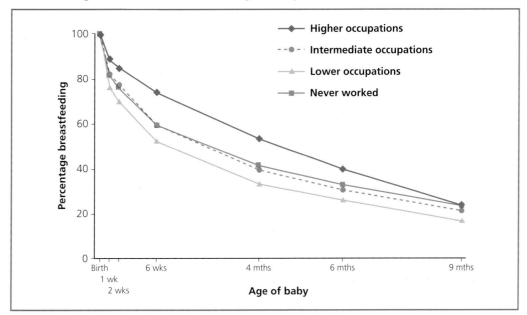

Age at which mother completed full-time education

Table 2.21 shows that in 2000, as in previous years, duration of breastfeeding was longest among mothers who continued in full-time education beyond the age of 18 and shortest among those who left school at 16 or below. For example, at six weeks, 78% of mothers who were educated beyond the age of 18 and who breastfed initially were still breastfeeding; this compares with 52% of mothers who left school at 16. Similar differentials can be seen at four, six and nine months.

Table 2.21

Table 2.21
Duration of breastfeeding for those who were breastfed initially by age mother left full-time education (United Kingdom, 2000)

	16 or under	17 or 18	Over 18	All babies**
	Percentage still breastfeeding			
Birth	100	100	100	100
1 week	77	82	91	84
2 weeks	71	77	88	79
6 weeks	52	60	78	64
4 months (17 weeks)	32	39	60	44
6 months (26 weeks)	24	29	47	34
9 months (39 weeks)*	13	16	27	19
Base (all Stage 3 mothers breastfeeding initially)	*1354*	*1794*	*1835*	*5023*

* Based on a reduced of cases excluding those babies who had not reached this age by Stage 3
** Includes some cases where mother's education not known

Ethnicity

White mothers who breastfed initially continued to do so for a shorter duration compared with mothers from other ethnic groups. Black mothers and those with mixed or other ethnic backgrounds breastfed the longest, being more likely than others to still be breastfeeding at all ages until 6 months.

Table 2.22, Figure 2.10

Table 2.22
Duration of breastfeeding for those who were breastfed initially by ethnic group
(United Kingdom, 2000)

	White	Asian	Black	Mixed & other**	All mothers
			Percentage still breastfeeding		
Birth	100	100	100	100	100
1 week	84	92	94	88	84
2 weeks	79	86	94	86	79
6 weeks	64	69	86	78	64
4 months (17 weeks)	44	43	61	61	44
6 months (26 weeks)	34	36	44	56	34
9 months (39 weeks)*	21	31	31	39	19
Base (all Stage 3 mothers breastfeeding initially)	*4586*	*132*	*97*	*93*	*5023*

* Based on a reduced number of cases excluding those babies who had not reached this age by Stage 3
** Includes some cases where ethnicity of mother not known
† Categories combined due to small base sizes

Figure 2.10
Duration of breastfeeding for those who were breastfed initially by ethnicity :
United Kingdom, 2000

Base: All Stage 3 mothers breastfeeding initially

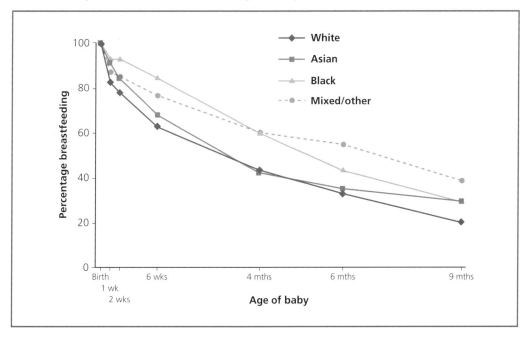

Mother's employment status

As in 1995, mothers were classified according to their working status during the first eight to nine months of their baby's life. Thus only mothers who completed all three stages of the survey are included in this analysis. Mother's were classified into one of five groups as follows:

i. those who were working when the baby was about six weeks old and continued working throughout the rest of the nine or so months ('working all the time' in Table 2.23);

ii. those who returned to work when the baby was between six weeks and four months old ('went back to work by Stage 2');

iii. those who returned to work when the baby was between four months and nine months old ('went back to work by Stage 3');

iv. those who did not work at all during the first nine or so months ('not working any of the time');

v. those whose pattern of work followed some other arrangement ('others').

Table 2.23 shows that the small group of mothers who did not give up work at all after the birth of their baby breastfed the longest; a half were still breastfeeding at 6 months, much higher than any other subgroup. As would be expected, among those who took a break before returning to work, the duration of breastfeeding was shorter for those who took a shorter break. Just over a third (37%) of women who returned to work by Stage 2 were still breastfeeding at 4 months compared with 53% of women who returned to work later.

Table 2.23

Table 2.23
Duration of breastfeeding for those who were breastfed initially by mother's working status during the first 9 months (UK, 2000)

	Working all the time	Went back to work by Stage 2	Went back to work by Stage 3	Not working any of the time	Others	All babies
	Percentage still breastfeeding					
Birth	100	100	100	100	100	100
1 week	91	81	88	84	76	84
2 weeks	86	76	85	79	72	79
6 weeks	68	60	72	64	54	64
4 months (17 weeks)	42	37	53	46	35	44
6 months (26 weeks)	53	25	38	39	25	34
9 months (39 weeks)*	23	11	16	26	11	19
Base (all Stage 3 mothers breastfeeding initially)	170	1131	1286	2196	240	5023

* Based on a reduced of cases excluding those babies who had not reached this age by Stage 3

2.5   Mixed breast and formula milk feeding

The tables and figures presented in this chapter so far show the proportion of mothers breastfeeding at different ages. However, these mothers may also be giving formula or cow's milk. In recent years there has been increasing interest in the level of women who breastfeed their child **exclusively.**

Infants are considered to be **exclusively breastfed** when they receive only breast milk, and no other food or drink with the exception of medicine, vitamins or mineral supplements (WHO 1991).

In the 2000 survey, we were unable to analyse information on exclusive breastfeeding as defined above. However, we were able to obtain data on how mothers were giving their milk feeds - whether wholly from the breast or in conjunction with other milk, such as formula. In this survey we use the term **"giving milk only from the breast"** which refers to **breastfeeding mothers who are not supplementing their baby's milk feeds with any formula or cows' milk.** However they may have been feeding their baby solids or giving them water or additional non-milk drinks.

Unfortunately, it is not possible to use the information collected in the survey to look at the prevalence of mothers giving only breastmilk at different ages, although we do know the status of mother's feeding **at the time they completed the questionnaire.** However, this information in itself is not very useful as there is such a wide variation in babies' ages at each stage, and the age ranges for each stage overlap to a certain extent (see Table 2.25). Thus, as a proxy for looking at prevalence of mothers giving only breastmilk at different ages, we have analysed the milk feeding practices by the age of baby at the time of completing the questionnaire.   Table 2.24 shows the results based on all mothers. For each age group a mean baby's age is given to facilitate interpretation of the data.

Although the analysis is rather crude, the data does give some indication of the prevalence of mothers giving breastmilk only and those giving mixed milk feeds at different ages. The data suggests that around three in ten mothers (29%) were giving milk only from the breast at approximately five weeks, this figure falling to one in five (20%) by around nine weeks. By approximately six months, only one in ten mothers (10%) were breastfeeding solely, this figure falling to 4% by around eleven months.

The data would suggest that the practice of giving milk only from the breast is more common than mixed milk feeding in the early stages, with around twice as many babies in the 3-6 week age group receiving only breastmilk than receiving mixed milk feeds. This gap then narrows, and the data suggests that from around seven months, an equal proportion of women are choosing to give mixed milk feeds as are giving milk only from the breast.

Table 2.24

Table 2.26

Milk feeding status at the three stages of survey by mother's socio-economic classification (NS-SEC) (United Kingdom 2000)

	Higher occupations	Intermed-iate occu-pations	Lower occupat-ions	Never occupat-ions	Unclass-ified	All mothers
	%	%	%	%	%	%
Breast milk only at Stage 1	38	26	18	14	21	25
Breast and other milk at Stage 1	23	17	12	15	19	17
Other milk only at Stage 1	39	57	70	71	60	58
Breast milk only at Stage 2	20	15	10	10	14	14
Breast and other milk at Stage 2	21	12	6	7	9	12
Other milk only at Stage 2	59	73	84	83	77	74
Breast milk only at Stage 3	7	8	5	5	7	6
Breast and other milk at Stage 3	11	6	4	5	7	7
Other milk only at Stage 3	82	86	91	90	86	87
Bases						
Stage 1 babies	*2790*	*1907*	*2619*	*1277*	*902*	*9492*
Stage 2 babies	*2545*	*1740*	*2286*	*979*	*750*	*8299*
Stage 3 babies	*2314*	*1558*	*1982*	*769*	*643*	*7267*
Means age of baby (days)						
Stage 1 babies	*47*	*48*	*47*	*50*	*49*	*48*
Stage 2 babies	*138*	*140*	*140*	*140*	*139*	*139*
Stage 3 babies	*277*	*275*	*276*	*276*	*274*	*276*

Figure 2.11

Milk feeding status at the three stages of the survey by mother's socio-economic classification: United Kingdom 2000

Base: All mothers at relevant stage

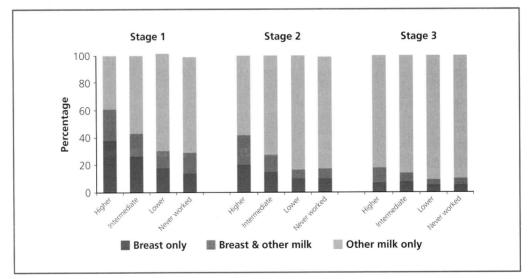

Table 2.27
Milk feeding status at the three stages of survey by ethnicity (United Kingdom 2000)

	White	Asian	Black	Mixed	Other	All mothers
	%	%	%	%	%	%
Breast milk only at Stage 1	25	24	28	35	33	25
Breast and other milk at Stage 1	15	37	51	26	30	17
Other milk only at Stage 1	60	39	21	39	37	58
Breast milk only at Stage 2	14	17	21	26	32	14
Breast and other milk at Stage 2	12	16	25	10	21	12
Other milk only at Stage 2	74	67	54	64	47	74
Breast milk only at Stage 3	6	9	7	18	[18]	6
Breast and other milk at Stage 3	6	8	17	12	[27]	7
Other milk only at Stage 3	88	83	76	70	[55]	87
Bases						
Stage 1 babies	8608	274	185	92	67	9492
Stage 2 babies	7632	202	132	80	57	8299
Stage 3 babies	6763	149	104	61	[44]	7267
Means age of baby (days)						
Stage 1 babies	47	54	54	47	53	48
Stage 2 babies	139	145	137	131	149	139
Stage 3 babies	276	279	271	275	281	276

* Total bases include some cases where ethnicity of mother not known

Figure 2.12
Milk feeding status at the three stages of the survey by ethnicity: United Kingdom 2000

Base: All mothers at relevant stage

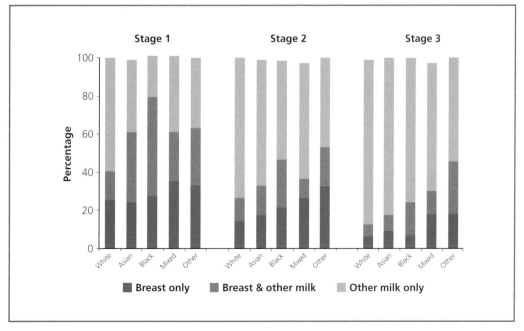

Age at which mother completed full-time education

There is a strong relationship between the milk feeding status of mothers and educational level. Mothers in the highest educational category were more likely to breastfeed either alone or in conjunction with other milk than women in the lower educational categories. However, the balance between sole breastfeeding and mixed milk feeding remains similar for the different subgroups at each stage.

Table 2.28, Figure 2.13

Table 2.28
Milk feeding status at the three stages of survey by age mother completed full-time education (United Kingdom 2000)

	16 or under	17 or 18	19+	All mothers
	%	%	%	%
Breast milk only at Stage 1	15	24	40	25
Breast and other milk at Stage 1	10	17	26	17
Other milk only at Stage 1	75	59	34	58
Breast milk only at Stage 2	8	13	24	14
Breast and other milk at Stage 2	6	11	21	12
Other milk only at Stage 2	86	76	55	74
Breast milk only at Stage 3	4	6	10	6
Breast and other milk at Stage 3	3	6	13	7
Other milk only at Stage 3	93	88	77	87
Bases*				
Stage 1 babies	*3436*	*3289*	*2683*	*9492*
Stage 2 babies	*2941*	*2915*	*2374*	*8299*
Stage 3 babies	*2510*	*2596*	*2104*	*7267*
Mean age of baby (days)				
Stage 1 babies	*48*	*47*	*49*	*48*
Stage 2 babies	*140*	*140*	*137*	*139*
Stage 3 babies	*277*	*276*	*276*	*276*

* Total bases include some cases where ethnicity of mother not known

Figure 2.13

Milk feeding status at the three stages of the survey by age mother completed full-time education: United Kingdom 2000

Base: All mothers at relevant stage

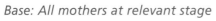

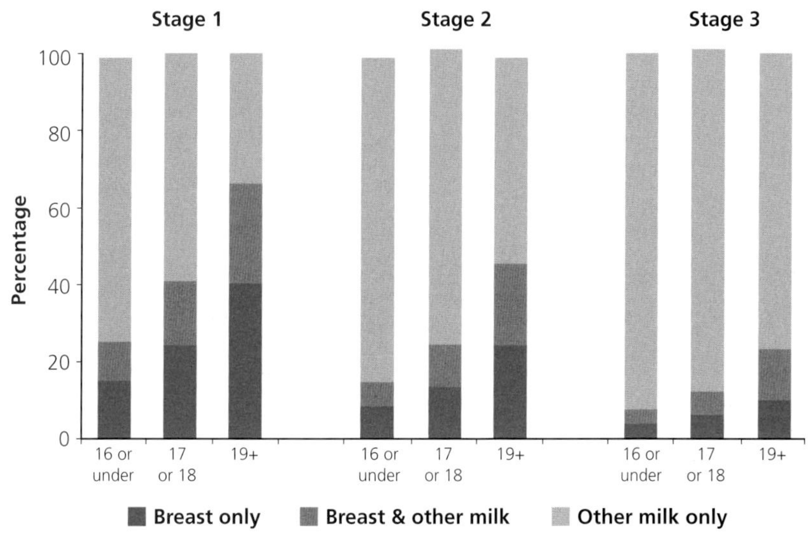

[1] Foster K, Lader D, Cheeseborough S Infant Feeding 1995, HMSO (London, 1997)

3

The use of milk other than breast milk

Summary

- In 2000, 30% of mothers in the United Kingdom did not breastfeed at all and gave infant formula as the sole source of nutrition from birth. This compares to 34% in 1995.
- By the first stage of the survey, when the babies were around four to ten weeks old, almost six in ten (58%) had switched entirely to infant formula milk. Some breastfeeding mothers were also using infant formula making a total of three-quarters of mothers who were using infant formula milk at least to some extent at the first stage of the survey.
- When babies were 4-10 weeks old, almost two-thirds (64%) of bottle feeding mothers were giving a whey dominant formula. At 4 – 5 months old, four in ten bottle feeding mothers (41%) were using a whey dominant formula and over a half (53%) a casein dominant one. At 8 – 9 months old, a fifth (20%) of bottle feeding mothers were using whey dominant and three in ten (30%) casein dominant formula. Over a third (37%) were using follow-on formula milk at this stage, a significant increase from 25% in 1995.
- At all three stages of the survey, breastfeeding mothers using formula milk were more likely to use a whey dominant formula than a casein dominant one. Breastfeeding mothers were also more likely than non-breastfeeding mothers to use a follow-on formula at stage three of the survey (49% compared with 36% amongst non-breastfeeding mothers).
- At stages one and two of the survey, less than 0.5% were giving cow's milk as a main milk drink. By stage three when the babies were 8 – 9 months old, 8% had introduced cow's milk as the main milk drink (down from 15% in 1995). Just under three in ten (28%) had introduced it as a secondary drink and just under half (47%) were using it to mix food. In total, 54% had introduced cow's milk to their baby in some way by stage three of the survey (61% in 1995).
- The vast majority of mothers giving their babies cow's milk as a drink were giving whole milk. Amongst mothers giving cow's milk as a drink, over eight in ten (84%) were giving whole milk, 15% were giving semi-skimmed milk and 1% skimmed milk.
- In 2000, under a quarter (23%) of first time mothers attending an antenatal class on feeding (12% of all first time mothers) were taught how to make up a bottle. In 1995, almost half (46%) of first time mothers attending such a class were shown how to do this.

This chapter is concerned with the use by mothers of milk other than breast milk, looking specifically at the type of formula milks given at the different stages, the use of cow's milk, mothers receiving help with the cost of milk and problems experienced by bottle-feeding mothers both in hospital and after leaving.

3.1 The use of infant formula milk

Infant formula milk is an artificial feed, manufactured to replace breast milk as a sole source of nutrition for babies until they are weaned. In the early stages of weaning, breast or infant formula milk continues to provide the majority of energy and nutrients for the baby.

In 2000, 30% of mothers in the United Kingdom did not breast feed at all and gave infant formula as the sole source of nutrition from birth. This compares to 34% in 1995. By the first stage of the survey, when the babies were around four to ten weeks old, almost six in ten - 58% - had switched entirely to infant formula milk (compared to 62% in 1995). So, around four in ten (39%) of those who breastfed their baby had given up this method of feeding in the early weeks. A further quarter (25%) of breastfeeding mothers were supplementing their breast milk with formula milk (27% in 1995). Thus in total, three-quarters of mothers were using infant formula milk at least to some extent by the time their baby was four to ten weeks old. Just a quarter of mothers were feeding their babies entirely with breast milk.

Table 3.1

Table 3.1

Feeding method at around 4 to 10 weeks (stage 1) by initial feeding method (United Kingdom 2000)

	Initial feeding method		All babies
	Breastfed at birth %	Not breastfed at birth %	%
Breastmilk only	36	-	25
Breastmilk & infant formula	25	-	17
Giving infant formula exclusively	39	100	58
Base (All stage 1 mothers)	*6561*	*2931*	*9492*

As noted above, a quarter of mothers were giving only breastmilk at stage 1 but around one in six were breastfeeding and giving infant formula at least to some extent: at this stage of the survey, 41% of breastfeeding mothers were also giving infant formula. This is a lower proportion than in 1995 when 46% of breastfeeding mothers were supplementing with infant formula at stage one of the survey, and halts the steady increase that had been seen in this proportion since 1985. However, it should be borne in mind that the babies at stage one of the survey were a little younger than in 1995 and this might partly explain this.

By the second stage of the survey, when the babies were around 4 – 5 months old, 45% of breastfeeding mothers were also giving their babies formula milk. This is a very similar proportion to that noted in 1995.

Table 3.2

Table 3.2
Milk other than breast milk given to breastfed babies at stages 1 and 2 (1995 and 2000, United Kingdom)

	Stage 1 (4-10 weeks)		Stage 2 (4-5 months)	
Milk given	**1995** **%**	**2000** **%**	**1995** **%**	**2000** **%**
Milk other than breast milk given	46	41	43	45
Only breast milk given	54	59	57	55
Base (Breastfeeding mothers)	*1954*	*4004*	*1236*	*2195*

There was some difference by country in the proportion of breastfeeding mothers also giving infant formula. As in 1995, at stage one of the survey, breastfeeding mothers in Scotland were least likely to supplement breast milk with infant formula and those in Northern Ireland most likely to do so. By stage two of the survey, when the babies were 4 – 5 months old, these differences were no longer apparent.

Table 3.3

Table 3.3
Milk other than breast milk given to breastfed babies at stages 1 and 2 by country (2000)

	Stage 1				Stage 2			
	England & Wales **%**	**Scotland** **%**	**Northern Ireland** **%**	**United Kingdom** **%**	**England & Wales** **%**	**Scotland** **%**	**Northern Ireland** **%**	**United Kingdom** **%**
Milk other than breast given	41	35	44	41	46	44	42	45
Only breast milk given	59	65	56	59	54	56	58	55
Base: Breastfeeding mothers	*2370*	*893*	*422*	*4004*	*1289*	*518*	*211*	*2195*

3.2   The different types of infant formula

The majority of infant formulas are based on cow's milk and can be classified according to the dominant cow's milk protein of either whey or casein. Casein dominant formulas are based on whole cow milk protein and have a casein:whey ratio of approximately 80:20. Whey dominant formulas are modified so that the casein:whey ratio is approximately

40:60, which is closer to that in breast milk. Some manufacturers claim that casein dominant formulas are more satisfying for older or hungrier babies. Although there is no firm evidence of this, these claims are likely to influence mothers.

Although most formulas are manufactured from cow's milk, some are available based on soy protein isolate as a protein source. These products may be used from birth but should not usually be a first choice unless there is a specific reason for excluding cow's milk products from the diet (COMA) [1].

Follow-on formulas, which are again based on cow's milk, may be used by mothers to provide the milk drink element in mixed diets of older babies. They are not intended to be used as a sole source of nutrition and the report of the COMA Working Group on the Weaning Diet recommends that follow-on milk should not be used as a replacement for breast milk or infant formula before the age of about six months.

The COMA report also recommends that whole cow's milk should only be used as a main milk drink after the age of one year. In addition, semi-skimmed milk is not suitable as a drink before the age of two years and fully skimmed cow's milk should not be introduced before the age of five years.

All mothers not giving only breastmilk were asked which types of milk they gave to their baby most of the time. For infant formula milk they were presented with a full list of brands from which to select their answer(s), and they were also asked to indicate which type of cow's milk they gave to their baby, if any. In analysis, the infant formula milks were coded as being whey or casein dominant.

As shown in Table 3.4 below, almost two-thirds (64%) of bottle feeding mothers were giving a whey dominant formula at stage one of the survey when the babies were 4 – 10 weeks old. This is an increase on the six in ten (60%) giving this type of formula in 1995, with a consequent decrease in the proportions using casein dominant formula from four in ten (38%) to a third (34%). However, by stage two of the survey, when the babies were 4 – 5 months old, around four in ten were using a whey dominant formula and over a half were using a casein dominant formula – similar to the picture in 1995. At stage three of the survey, when the babies were 8 – 9 months, around a fifth were giving a whey dominant formula and three in ten a casein dominant formula.

At all three stages only a very small minority were using a soya based formula (1 – 2% of mothers giving milk other than breast milk). At stages one and two, only a very small number of mothers were giving any form of cows milk (fewer than 0.5%), though this rose to almost one in ten mothers by stage three (9%). None of the mothers said they gave skimmed cows milk most of the time and almost all the mothers giving cows milk at stage three indicated that this was whole milk. Since 1985, there has been a big change in the use of cow's milk – 7% were using it at stage two of the survey in 1985, down to 1% by 1995, and in 2000 an insignificant number of mothers were giving cows milk at stage two and less than 10% at stage three – a decline from the 16% using it in 1995.

The greatest change in use of milk other than breast milk since 1995 is in the use of follow-on formula at stage three of the survey when the babies were 8 – 9 months old. This was a trend noted in 1995, when a quarter of mothers giving milk other than from the breast were using follow-on formula (up from 5% in 1990). By 2000 this had risen to well over a third (37%), predominantly as in 1995 due to a fall in the proportions giving cow's milk.

Table 3.4

Table 3.4
Main type of milk other than breast milk given by mothers (1995 and 2000 United Kingdom)

	Stage 1		Stage 2		Stage 3	
	1995 %	2000 %	1995 %	2000 %	1995 %	2000 %
Whey dominant	60	64	39	41	22	20
Casein dominant	38	34	54	53	33	30
Soya-based formula	} 2	1	2	2	3	2
Follow-on formula		*	2	4	25	37
Cows milk	*	*	1	*	16	9
– Whole	*	*	1	*	14	9
– Semi-skimmed	*	*	*	*	1	–
– Skimmed	–	–	*	–	*	–
Other/inadequately described	1	1	1	1	1	2
Base (Mothers giving milk other than breast milk)	*4076*	*5991*	*4461*	*7102*	*4826*	*6690*

There were some differences in the choice of type of milk between mothers who were also breastfeeding and those who were not. Breastfeeding mothers were more likely to choose a whey rather than casein based formula at all three stages of the survey: 85% of them did so at stage one, 65% at stage two and 22% at stage three (comparative figures for 1995 are only available for Great Britain rather than the UK, when 82% of mothers combining breast and formula milk gave a whey based formula at stage one, 70% gave this at stage two and 27% at stage three). At stage three, breastfeeding mothers were more likely than non- breastfeeding mothers to be using follow-on formula milk (49% of them using this type of milk compared with 36% of non-breastfeeding mothers). Both groups of mothers were equally likely to be using cows milk – a change from the position in 1995 when breastfeeding mothers were more likely than non-breastfeeding mothers to be giving cows milk at stage three of the survey (26% of breastfeeding mothers and 15% of non-breastfeeding mothers in Great Britain).

Table 3.5, Figure 3.1

There were also differences in the types of milk used between the countries. As in 1995, mothers in England and Wales were more likely than those in Scotland and Northern Ireland to use a whey rather than casein based formula, with mothers in Scotland and Northern Ireland being more likely than those in England and Wales to use a casein based formula. By stage three of the survey, when the babies were 8 – 9 months old, mothers in England and Wales were more likely than those in Scotland and Northern Ireland to give follow-on formula, with these latter two groups being more likely to give cow's milk than mothers in England and Wales. There has however been a decrease in the use of cow's milk since 1995 in all countries (from 15% to 8% in England and Wales, 21% to 12% in Scotland and 23% to 15% in Northern Ireland).

Table 3.6

Table 3.5

Main type of milk other than breast milk given at each stage by whether mothers were also breastfeeding (United Kingdom 2000)

	Mothers not breastfeeding at:			Mothers who were also breastfeeding at:		
	Stage 1 %	Stage 2 %	Stage 3 %	Stage 1 %	Stage 2 %	Stage 3 %
Whey dominant	62	37	20	85	65	22
Casein dominant	36	57	31	12	30	13
Soya-based formula	1	1	2	1	2	2
Follow-on formula	*	4	36	–	3	49
Cows milk	*	*	9	*	*	9
Other/inadequately described	1	1	2	1	*	5
Base (Mothers giving milk other than breast milk)	5415	6033	6212	576	966	470

Figure 3.1

Main type of milk other than breast milk given at each stage by whether mothers were also breastfeeding (United Kingdom 2000)

Base: Mothers giving milk other than breastmilk

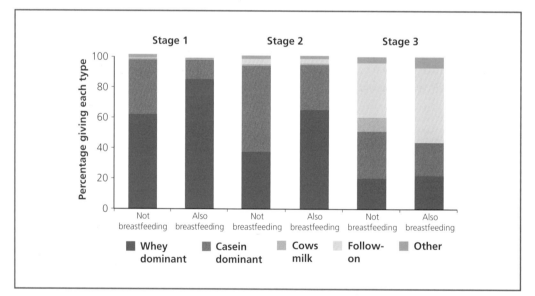

Table 3.6
Main type of milk other than breast milk given at each stage by country (2000)

	Stage 1 (4 – 10 weeks)			Stage 2 (4 – 5 months)			Stage 3 (8 – 9 months)		
	England & Wales %	Scotland %	Northern Ireland %	England & Wales %	Scotland %	Northern Ireland %	England & Wales %	Scotland %	Northern Ireland %
Whey dominant	67	52	49	42	33	26	21	16	15
Casein dominant	32	46	47	52	61	61	29	35	35
Soya-based formula	1	1	1	2	1	2	2	2	4
Follow-on formula	*	*	–	3	4	5	38	33	27
Cows milk	*	–	–	*	*	*	8	12	15
Other/inadequately described	1	*	2	1	1	2	2	2	3
Base (Mothers giving non-breast milk)	*3399*	*1488*	*1401*	*4010*	*1655*	*1491*	*3775*	*1598*	*1368*

Use of ready-to-feed infant formula

Infant formula milk has long been available as dry powder to be reconstituted with water but, for over ten years, ready-to-feed milk has also been obtainable. All mothers who were using infant formula milk were asked at all three stages of the survey whether they used ready-to-feed milk.

Around one in eight (12%) mothers giving formula milk indicated that they used ready-to-feed milk at stage one, dropping to one in ten at stage two and rising a little to one in eight at stage three of the survey.

Table 3.7

Table 3.7
Use of powdered and ready to feed infant formula (United Kingdom, 2000)

	Stage 1 %	Stage 2 %	Stage 3 %
Powdered	80	82	86
Ready to Feed	3	2	3
Both	9	8	10
Base (All mothers giving formula milk)	*5984*	*7051*	*6102*

Although only used by the minority, this is a significant increase on the proportions using ready-to-feed in 1995, when the proportions varied between 3% and 6%. As in 1995, mothers who were breastfeeding were more likely to use ready-to-feed milk than those giving only formula milk, particularly at stage one of the survey when the babies were young: as many as a quarter of breastfeeding mothers also gave ready-to-feed milk when their babies were four to ten weeks old.

Table 3.8

Table 3.8

The use of ready-to feed infant formulas at different stages (1995 Great Britain and 2000 United Kingdom)*

	Stage 1		Stage 2		Stage 3	
	1995 %	2000 %	1995 %	2000 %	1995 %	2000 %
Mothers not breastfeeding	4	10	4	9	3	13
Mothers who were also breastfeeding	13	25	10	16	5	20
All mothers giving formula milk	**6**	**12**	**4**	**10**	**3**	**13**
Bases:						
Mothers not breastfeeding	*3057*	*5409*	*3780*	*6055*	*4325*	*5675*
Mothers who were also breastfeeding	*872*	*575*	*529*	*996*	*315*	*427*
All mothers giving formula milk	***3930***	***5984***	***4300***	***7051***	***4639***	***6102***

* Note that 1995 figures based on GB, 2000 on UK

There was some variation in use of ready-to-feed milk by country. At the first two stages, mothers in England and Wales were most likely to use it and those in Northern Ireland were least likely to do so. By stage three, when the babies were 8 – 9 months old, these differences were less apparent.

Table 3.9

Table 3.9

The use of ready-to feed infant formulas at different stages by country (2000)

	Stage 1			Stage 2			Stage 3		
	England & Wales %	Scotland %	Northern Ireland %	England & Wales %	Scotland %	Northern Ireland %	England & Wales %	Scotland %	Northern Ireland %
Ready-to-feed only	3	2	2	2	1	1	3	2	3
Ready-to-feed & powdered	9	8	5	9	8	5	10	11	8
All using ready to feed	**12**	**10**	**7**	**11**	**9**	**6**	**13**	**13**	**11**
Base (Mothers giving formula milk)	*3343*	*1467*	*1351*	*3883*	*1606*	*1406*	*3409*	*1380*	*1116*

Additions to formula

Mothers giving formula milk were asked whether they ever added anything to the milk. Only a minority did so (ranging from 5% at stage one to 6% at stages two and three). What they added varied. At all three stages less than 0.5% of bottle feeding mothers added sugar or honey to the milk. At stage one, colic drops and gripe water were most commonly added but still by only 1% of bottle feeding mothers in each case. At stages two and three mothers were most likely to add something to thicken the milk, such as rusks or baby rice but again only 1% of mothers giving a bottle did this.

3.3   Choice of brand of formula

The infant formula that a mother uses may be influenced by the brand first used, which for most mothers bottle feeding from birth will be that used while they were in hospital. All mothers giving infant formula from birth were therefore asked if they were offered any choice of brand while in hospital. Just under nine in ten (87%) said that they were, a slight fall from the 92% of the comparable group of mothers who gave this answer in 1995. Mothers in Scotland were a little less likely to say they had been offered a choice.

Table 3.10

Table 3.10
Whether mothers were given a choice of infant formula in hospital by country (2000)

	England & Wales	Scotland	Northern Ireland	United Kingdom
	%	%	%	%
Mother given a choice	87	84	88	87
Mother not given a choice	13	16	12	13
Base: Stage 1 mothers giving infant formula from birth	2321	1097	1004	4156

Since leaving hospital, only three in ten mothers (30% in the United Kingdom, 29% in Great Britain) said they had changed brand after leaving hospital. This continues the downward trend noted since 1985 – in 1985 44% of bottle feeding mothers in Great Britain had changed brands at stage one of the survey and by 1995 this had decreased to 35%.

As in previous years, the most common reason for changing the formula used was because the mother thought the baby was still hungry or not satisfied (70%). Other reasons given included the baby being sick (15%), constipated (11%) or having an allergy (3%). One in twenty mothers who had changed brands did so because they preferred a different brand from that given in hospital. Included in other answers given were changing brands due to colic (2%) or unavailability (2%), or on the advice of the health visitor (1%).

Table 3.11

As in 1995, mothers in Scotland and Northern Ireland were more likely to change their brand of milk due to believing their babies to be hungry. This could account for mothers in these two countries being more likely than those in England and Wales to use casein dominant formula milk.

Table 3.12

Table 3.17

Where mothers usually exchanged milk tokens at stage 1, by country (2000)

	England & Wales	Scotland	Northern Ireland	United Kingdom
	%	%	%	%
Child health clinic	71	71	51	69
With the milkman	11	5	17	11
At a supermarket	20	15	6	19
At another type of shop	14	21	28	16
Somewhere else/not stated	7	9	14	8
Base: All Stage 1 mothers who received tokens	*912*	*407*	*430*	*1638*

Percentages do not add up to 100 as some mothers exchanged at more than one place

Mothers only giving breastmilk were most likely to exchange their tokens at the supermarket. This is presumably because they were exchanging them for cow's milk for themselves, which is more readily available in supermarkets than at the child health clinic. A quarter used them at the child health clinic. A fifth exchanged them with the milkman – a decrease from the 47% of breastfeeding mothers receiving tokens who exchanged them with the milkman in 1995.

In contrast, over three quarters of mothers giving only formula milk exchanged their tokens at the child health clinic; just under a fifth took them to the supermarket and one in ten exchanged them with the milkman.

Table 3.18

Table 3.18

Where mothers usually exchanged milk tokens at stage 1, by feeding method (United Kingdom, 2000)

	Breastfed	Breast & other milk	Not breastfed	Total
	%	%	%	%
Child health clinic	25	60	77	69
With the milkman	20	12	9	11
At a supermarket	46	26	14	19
At another type of shop	22	14	15	16
Somewhere else/not stated	2	3	3	3
Base: All Stage 1 mothers who received tokens	*205*	*121*	*1304*	*1638*

Percentages do not add up to 100 as some mothers exchanged at more than one place
* Includes some mothers for whom feeding method not known

3.6 Problems with giving manufactured baby milk

In 2000, as in previous years, mothers who did not breast feed were less likely to report feeding problems than mothers who did. However, bottle feeding mothers did experience some problems, as described below.

The majority of mothers will use infant formula at some stage, so at stage one of the survey, mothers were asked if they had been shown at their antenatal class (if they attended) how to make up a bottle. This issue is mainly relevant to first time mothers.

In 2000 almost two thirds (64%) of first time mothers attended antenatal classes. The vast majority of them (52% of all first time mothers) had attended a talk on feeding their baby although less than a quarter of this subgroup (12% of all first time mothers) were shown how to make up a bottle. This compares with just over a quarter of first time mothers (27%) being shown how to make up a bottle in 1995. In 1995, 46% of first time mothers attending a class on feeding were shown how to make up a bottle. In 2000, the equivalent percentage was 23%.

Amongst those attending classes, those intending to bottle feed were more likely to be shown how to make up a bottle, but as breast feeding mothers were more likely to attend classes in the first place, a higher proportion of breastfeeding first time mothers than bottle feeding first time mothers were shown how to make up a bottle at antenatal classes (13% compared with 9%).

Table 3.19

Table 3.19
Sources of information on infant feeding for mothers of first babies by intended feeding method (United Kingdom, 2000)

| | Intended feeding method | | | |
| | Infant formula | Breast* | Not decided | Total** |
	%	%	%	%
Attended antenatal classes	39	74	56	64
Attended a talk on feeding at a class	26	61	43	52
Taught how to make up a bottle at a class	9	13	9	12
Base: All Stage 1 mothers of first babies	922	3112	390	4448

* Including those intending to give breast & formula
** Includes some mothers for whom feeding intentions not recorded

Problems giving infant formula from a bottle in hospital

Compared with 1990 and 1995, fewer mothers who bottle fed from birth experienced problems bottle feeding while in hospital. One in eight (13%) of mothers who bottle fed from birth in the United Kingdom - compared with 17% in 1995 – said they had experienced problems. As in previous years, mothers of first babies were more likely to encounter problems than mothers of second or later children (16% compared with 11%).

A variety of problems were mentioned, as shown in table 3.20 below. Around a fifth in each case mentioned that either the baby was vomiting or, probably more seriously, that the baby had to be fed by tube. One in six mothers of first babies said their baby rejected the bottle – though only about a third of this percentage of mothers of second or later babies (6%) had this problem. Other problems mentioned were that the baby would not suck, was too slow feeding, would fall asleep during feeds, was in special care, hungry, and had colic or wind.

Table 3.20

Table 3.20
Feeding problems reported by mothers who used infant formula from birth by birth order (United Kingdom 2000)

	First births	Later births	All births
	%	%	%
Baby:			
Vomiting	20	24	22
Fed by tube	17	23	20
Wouldn't feed from bottle	17	6	11
Wouldn't suck	7	11	9
Fed too slowly	4	10	7
Always falling asleep	9	5	7
In special care	2	8	5
Hungry	5	4	4
Had colic/wind	7	2	4
Had other problems	17	23	21
Problem not specified	5	13	9
Base (Stage 1 mothers using infant formula from birth & having feeding problems)	*171*	*187*	*358*

Mothers who had problems feeding their baby formula milk were asked whether or not they were able to get help in the hospital. Around nine in ten (85%) said they were, the majority receiving help from a midwife (59%) or nurse (41%). Just under a fifth (18%) received help from a doctor (18%), though first time mothers were less likely to remember being helped by a doctor than second-time or later mothers.

Table 3.21

Problems giving infant formula from a bottle at home

Just under four in ten of mothers (39%) were exclusively giving infant formula when they left hospital and a further 8% of mothers were combining breast and bottle feeding. Amongst these mothers, 14% said they had experienced problems feeding their baby since they returned home. This compares with 17% in 1995. Many different types of problems were mentioned, as shown in table 3.22. Over a quarter of mothers giving infant formula believed their babies had been hungry and not satisfied – first time mothers were particularly likely to believe this had been the case. Over a fifth mentioned that their baby had wind or colic and one in six reported that their baby had been vomiting. A number of mothers giving formula milk reported that they had problems breastfeeding, with getting the baby to latch on, not having enough breast milk and having painful breasts. It could be hypothesised that these mothers turned to bottle feeding because they had these breastfeeding problems or that the breastfeeding problems were partly caused by trying to use a combined breast and bottle feeding method.

Table 3.22

Table 3.21
Source of advice for mothers experiencing problems with feeding infant formula in hospital by birth order (United Kingdom 2000)

	First births	Later births	All births
	%	%	%
Midwife	61	58	59
Nurse	46	37	41
Doctor	8	27	18
Friend/relative	8	3	6
Did not receive help/not stated	11	18	15
Base (Stage 1 mothers using infant formula from birth & having feeding problems)	*171*	*187*	*358*

Percentages do not add up to 100 as some mothers received advice from more than one source

Table 3.22
Feeding problems after leaving hospital amongst mothers giving infant formula from birth by birth order (United Kingdom 2000)

	First births	Later births	All births*
	%	%	%
Baby seemed hungry/not satisfied	33	23	28
Baby had wind/colic	23	21	22
Baby vomiting	15	19	17
Wouldn't latch on	11	10	10
Baby constipated	6	7	6
Not enough breastmilk/dried up	6	4	5
Painful breast/nipples/mastitis	5	4	4
Baby always falling asleep	2	6	4
Baby fed too slowly	2	6	4
Mother tired/ill	3	3	3
Baby wouldn't suck	2	3	2
Baby wouldn't feed from bottle	2	2	2
Baby not gaining weight	3	2	2
Baby didn't like bottle milk	1	2	2
Other problems	13	16	15
Base (Stage 1 mothers giving infant formula after hospital & having feeding problems after hospital)	*288*	*325*	*613*

* Includes mothers giving mixed breast and formula feeds

The vast majority of those giving formula milk after leaving hospital and experiencing feeding problems received professional advice. Just one in ten of this subgroup did not receive help. Six in ten received advice from a health visitor and almost half from a midwife. Just over a fifth were advised by a doctor or GP. A similar proportion turned to friends or relatives, first time mothers being particularly likely to do this.

Table 3.23

Table 3.23

Source of advice for mothers experiencing problems with feeding infant formula at home by birth order (United Kingdom 2000)

	First births	Later births	All births*
	%	%	%
Doctor/GP	18	25	22
Health visitor	62	61	61
Midwife	51	45	48
Nurse	2	6	4
Friend/relative	28	15	21
Books/leaflets/magazines	11	5	8
Other	2	4	3
Did not receive help	9	10	10
Base (Stage 1 mothers using infant formula from birth & having feeding problems after hospital)	*288*	*3255*	*613*

Percentages do not add up to 100 as some mothers received advice from more than one source

* Includes mothers giving mixed breast and formula feeds

[1] Weaning and the Weaning Diet. Report of the Working Group on the Weaning Diet of the Committee on the Medical Aspects of Food Policy. Department of Health. HMSO (London 1994)

4

Antenatal care, smoking and drinking

Summary

- Almost all mothers (98%) had antenatal check-ups during pregnancy. Almost two-thirds (64%) of mothers of first babies had been to antenatal classes; this was a significantly lower proportion than in 1995 when 70% of mothers of first babies attended antenatal classes.
- 92% of mothers knew that increasing their intake of folic acid in early pregnancy could be beneficial. In 1995, 75% were aware of this. Almost nine in ten (89%) of all mothers had increased their intake in early pregnancy. Almost three-quarters (73%) took supplements and three in ten (31%) changed their diet. Around one in six mothers did both.
- Just over half (54%) of mothers in the United Kingdom took supplementary iron or vitamins during pregnancy, this being significantly more common in Northern Ireland where 71% took supplements.
- Just over a third (35%) of mothers in the United Kingdom smoked in the twelve months before or during their pregnancy. Three percent gave up smoking less than a year before pregnancy and were still not smoking at stage one of the survey and a further 11% gave up on confirmation of pregnancy and stayed quit. A fifth (20%) of women in the UK smoked throughout their pregnancy, even if they cut down.
- 87% of mothers drank alcohol in the two years before they became pregnant. Six in ten (61%) drank during pregnancy, a decline on the position in 1995, when two-thirds (66%) drank during pregnancy. The majority of those drinking in pregnancy (71%) drank less than one unit per week on average.
- 86% of smokers received information on the effect of smoking during pregnancy. This is the same proportion as in 1995. 77% of women who drank received advice on the effect of alcohol. This was an increase on the 71% who received advice about alcohol in 1995.

In this chapter, we investigate the attendance of mothers at ante-natal check-ups and classes, knowledge about folic acid supplementation during pregnancy, and smoking and drinking behaviour of mothers before, during and after pregnancy.

4.1 Antenatal check-ups, classes and home visits

Almost all mothers (98%) had antenatal check-ups during pregnancy. As in 1995, the proportions were similar in all countries and for first and later births. In England and Wales, around a half were seen at home by a midwife in connection with their pregnancy and a small minority were visited by a health visitor before the birth. Mothers in Scotland were less likely than those in England and Wales to receive a home visit with just four in ten saying they had experienced this. This indicates a change from the position in 1995 when six in ten mothers in Scotland (61%) said they had been seen at home prior to the birth. In Northern Ireland, around a third of expectant mothers were visited at home by a midwife and one in twenty by a health visitor, again this representing a decline on the percentage visited at home in 1995 (37% versus 49% in 1995). In all countries, visits were equally likely for first and later births.

Mothers were asked if they had gone to any classes to prepare for having their baby and by whom the classes had been organised. Women in Scotland were most likely to have attended classes (46%, as in 1995) and those in Northern Ireland least likely (32%). In England and Wales, the proportion attending antenatal classes dropped significantly to 36% in 2000 from 41% in 1995. As would be expected, women expecting their first child were more likely to have been to classes than were women who already had children: in England and Wales the rates were 64% and 11% respectively.

Table 4.1

Table 4.1

Proportion of mothers who reported antenatal check-ups, classes and home visits by birth order and country (2000)

	England & Wales			Scotland			Northern Ireland			United Kingdom		
	First birth %	Later births %	All %	First birth %	Later births %	All %	First birth %	Later births %	All %	First birth %	Later births %	All %
Had antenatal check-ups	98	98	98	99	99	99	98	99	99	98	98	98
Went to antenatal classes	64	11	36	74	20	46	65	9	32	64	11	36
Had antenatal home visit:												
Midwife	49	48	49	28	32	30	34	31	32	47	46	47
Health visitor	7	6	7	13	8	11	6	4	5	7	6	7
Base (Stage 1 mothers)	*2560*	*2881*	*5441*	*1115*	*1159*	*2274*	*729*	*1049*	*1778*	*4448*	*5044*	*9492*

Attendance at antenatal classes was strongly associated with occupational group. Among mothers of first babies, 82% of mothers in higher occupations had been to classes compared with 54% of those in lower occupations and only 27% of those who had never worked or had been long term unemployed. A similar pattern was also seen for later births.

Table 4.2, Figure 4.1

Table 4.2
Proportion of mothers who went to antenatal classes by mother's socio-economic group (NS-SEC) and birth order (United Kingdom 2000)

	First births	Later births	All	First births	Later births	All
Percentage who went to antenatal classes						Bases
Higher occupations	82	18	51	1424	1367	2791
Intermediate occupations	76	13	42	898	1007	1905
Lower occupations	54	8	29	1200	1418	2618
Never worked	27	6	15	498	777	1275
Unclassified	56	11	32	427	474	901
All Stage 1 mothers	65	11	36	4448	5044	9492

Figure 4.1
Proportion of mothers of first babies who went to antenatal classes by mother's NS-SEC (2000, UK)
Base: All Stage 1 mothers

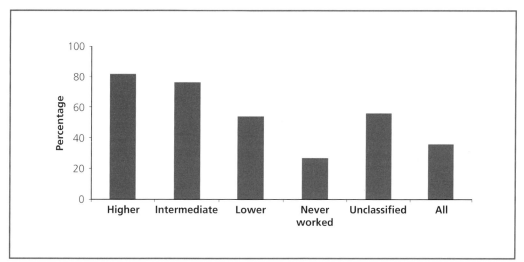

As in 1995, there was significant variation between countries in who had organised the antenatal classes. In Northern Ireland, women were most likely to have been to classes run by a hospital (70%) whereas in England and Wales they were more likely to be organised by a clinic, surgery or health centre (61%). Only a small proportion of women had been to classes run by a voluntary organisation and this was more common in England and Wales (9% of women who attended classes) than elsewhere (2% in Scotland and 1% in Northern Ireland).

Table 4.3

Table 4.3
Who organised antenatal classes by country (2000)

	England & Wales	Scotland	Northern Ireland	United Kingdom
	%	%	%	%
Hospital	40	51	70	42
Clinic/Surgery/Health Centre	61	55	33	59
Voluntary Organisation (e.g. NCT)	9	2	1	8
Other	3	1	1	3
Base (Stage 1 mothers who went to antenatal classes)	*1947*	*1052*	*566*	*3445*

Percentages do not add up to 100% as some mothers gave more than one answer

4.2 Folic acid and dietary supplements

In 1995, mothers were asked for the first time whether they knew that increasing their intake of folic acid could be good for them when they became pregnant. The Department of Health advises women to take a daily supplement of 400 micrograms of folic acid prior to conception and during the first twelve weeks of pregnancy and, in addition, to ensure that their diet is rich in foods containing folic acid.

In interpreting the results of this question it should be borne in mind that some mothers may have learned of the benefits of folic acid in the early weeks of their pregnancy when they had their first ante-natal appointment and their memory of when they first gained this information may be not entirely accurate. Nonetheless, the same would have been true in 1995 and what is interesting is any variation in the position since 1995 and any differences between subgroups of mothers in their knowledge and behaviour.

In 1995, three quarters (75%) of mothers in the United Kingdom said that they knew that increasing their intake of folic acid was good for them in early pregnancy. By 2000, this proportion had risen to over nine in ten (92%). Knowledge was almost universal in all subgroups though some mothers were a little better informed than others: for example, 98% of mothers in higher occupations were aware, compared with 93% of those in lower occupations.

Most women who knew about the benefits of folic acid also said they had taken some action to increase their intake. Three in ten (31%, up significantly from 26% in 1995) of all mothers had changed their diet and almost three-quarters (73%, up from 50% in 1995) had taken supplements; some had done both. However, there is no evidence of when mothers actually took this action, whether prior to conception or after they realised they were pregnant.

Compared with other countries, mothers in Scotland were more likely, and those in Northern Ireland least likely, to change their diet.

Table 4.4

Table 4.4
Action taken to increase intake of folic acid by country (2000)

	England & Wales	Scotland	Northern Ireland	United Kingdom
	%	%	%	%
Changed diet	31	34	28	31
Took supplements	73	74	74	73
No action taken	11	10	11	11
Base (All stage 1 mothers)	*5440*	*2274*	*1778*	*9492*

Percentages do not add up to 100% as some mothers gave more than one answer.

Looking more generally at dietary supplements, mothers were asked if they had taken any vitamin or iron supplements at all during pregnancy. Overall, just over half (54%) of mothers had done so and taking supplements was more common in Northern Ireland (71%), as it was in 1995.

As in 1995, most mothers who had taken supplements (93%) had taken iron, with just four in ten of this subgroup (39%) having taken vitamins. However, the percentage of all mothers taking vitamins has risen significantly since 1995 (from 15% to 21%), while the proportion of mothers taking iron during pregnancy has fallen significantly from six in ten (59%) to half (50%). This decrease has been particularly notable in Northern Ireland: in 1995, 82% of mothers in Northern Ireland supplemented their diet with iron; by 2000 this percentage had dropped to 70%. In England and Wales and Scotland in 2000, just under half (49%) of prospective mothers took iron, a significant drop of 8 and 5 percentage points respectively. These changes are as expected, given changes in practice in the prescription of iron over the last five years.

Table 4.5

Table 4.5
Type of supplements taken by country (2000)

	England & Wales	Scotland	Northern Ireland	United Kingdom
	%	%	%	%
Iron only	33	36	54	34
Vitamins only	5	4	3	5
Vitamins and iron	16	13	16	16
Other supplements	2	3	3	2
Base (All stage 1 mothers)	*5441*	*2274*	*1778*	*9492*

Percentages do not add up to 100% as some mothers gave more than one answer.

Although there is little variation by demographic subgroup, there is an indication that those educated for a longer period were more likely to take supplements: 61% of those who completed their education at the age of 18 or older took supplements, significantly higher than 50% of those with a terminal education age of 16 or less, and 53% of those who finished their full time education at age 17 or 18 years.

4.3   Smoking

At the first stage of the survey, when the babies were aged between about four and ten weeks, all mothers were asked a number of questions about smoking: if they had ever smoked, if they had smoked in the two years before the survey (since October 1998) and if they smoked now. They were also asked a series of questions about smoking in pregnancy and the smoking habits of the people with whom they lived. Some of these questions were similar to those asked in 1995 but many were revised to improve the reliability of the results. Therefore, only limited direct comparisons can be made with the 1995 results.

4.3.1   Smoking during pregnancy

Just over half (52%) of mothers in the United Kingdom said they had never smoked and a further 13% gave up smoking over a year before pregnancy. The remaining 35% of mothers smoked in the year before or during their pregnancy, although 3% gave up before their pregnancy was confirmed and were still not smoking at stage one of the survey. Just over one in ten (11%) gave up on confirmation of pregnancy and 1% gave up smoking later in pregnancy and stayed quit.

The remaining 20% of mothers in the United Kingdom smoked throughout their pregnancy, though most of these smokers did cut down and some did give up but then started again. Table 4.6 shows a full analysis of smoking behaviour by country, the mothers being allocated into mutually exclusive categories.

Table 4.6

The government has set a target for England in 'Smoking Kills - A White Paper on Tobacco' (1998) to reduce the proportion of women who continue to smoke during pregnancy to 15% by the year 2010, with a fall to 18% by 2005.

Table 4.7 summarises the percentages of women smoking before and throughout pregnancy by country. In 2000, 19% of women smoked throughout their pregnancy in England and in Wales. Results from the 1995 survey are not directly comparable due to the change in questions asked (see appendix 1), though results from that survey indicated that in England and Wales, 23% smoked throughout their pregnancy in 1995, while in Scotland 28% and in Northern Ireland, 27% did so.

This continues the downward trend noted since 1990 (in Great Britain in 1990, 28% of mothers smoked during pregnancy).

Table 4.7

Table 4.6
Smoking behaviour of all mothers by country (2000)

	United Kingdom	England	England & Wales	Scotland	Northern Ireland
	%	%	%	%	%
Non-smokers	**65**	**65**	**65**	**64**	**64**
Never smoked	52	52	52	53	54
Gave up smoking over a year before pregnancy	13	13	13	11	10
All smokers	**35**	**35**	**35**	**36**	**36**
Smoked before pregnancy but gave up	16	16	16	14	14
Gave up smoking less than a year before pregnancy	3	3	3	3	3
Gave up smoking on confirmation of pregnancy	11	11	11	9	10
Gave up later in pregnancy, stayed quit	2	2	2	2	1
Smoked throughout pregnancy	20	19†	19	22	23
Gave up, but started again	4	4	4	5	4
Cut down	14	14	14	15	16
Did not cut down	2	2	2	2	3
Base (All stage 1 mothers)*	*9126*	*4921*	*5225*	*2206*	*1722*

* Excluding 366 mothers for whom smoking status could not be classified
† The percentage for women smoking in England given in the first release of the data in August 2001 was 18%. This was based on preliminary data.

Table 4.7
Smoking and Pregnancy by country (2000)

	Percentage who smoked before or during pregnancy	Percentage who smoked throughout pregnancy	Base: All stage 1 mothers*	Percentage who gave up before or during pregnancy	Base:: Stage 1 mothers who smoked before or during pregnancy
	%	%		%	
England	35	19	*4921*	45	*1720*
England and Wales	35	19	*5225*	45	*1844*
Scotland	36	22	*2206*	39	*802*
Northern Ireland	36	23	*1722*	38	*625*
United Kingdom	35	20	*9126*	44	*3233*

*Excludes 366 mothers who did not supply sufficient information for classifying their smoking status.

It is well known from surveys such as the General Household Survey that there is a strong association between smoking and socio-economic classification and this pattern was also seen in this survey. Women in higher occupations were less likely than other mothers to have smoked either before or throughout their pregnancy and were more likely to have given up smoking during pregnancy. In the United Kingdom as a whole, 63% of mothers in higher occupations who had smoked in the year before pregnancy gave up smoking either before or during their pregnancy, compared with 38% of mothers in lower occupations and 29% of mothers who had never worked or were long term unemployed. Figure 4.2 illustrates this and Tables 4.8 - 4.12 give a detailed breakdown by country.

Tables 4.8–4.12, Figure 4.2

Figure 4.2
Prevalence of smoking before and throughout pregnancy by mother's NS-SEC (2000, UK)

Base: All Stage 1 mothers

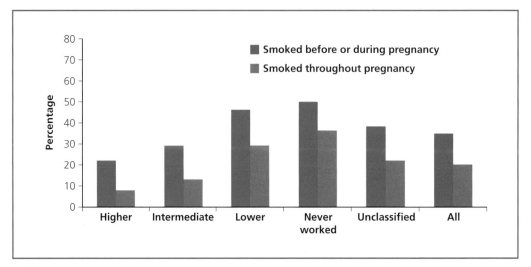

Table 4.8
Smoking and pregnancy by mother's socio-economic group (NS-SEC) (United Kingdom 2000)

	Percentage who smoked before or during pregnancy	Percentage who smoked throughout pregnancy	Base: All stage 1 mothers*	Percentage who gave up before or during pregnancy	Base:: Stage 1 mothers who smoked before or during pregnancy
	%	%		%	
Higher occupations	22	8	2684	63	589
Intermediate occupations	29	13	1837	55	531
Lower occupations	46	29	2510	38	1164
Never worked	50	36	1233	29	617
Unclassified	38	22	863	43	332
All mothers	**35**	**20**	**9126**	**44**	**3233**

*Excludes 366 mothers who did not supply sufficient information for classifying their smoking status.

Table 4.9

Smoking and pregnancy in England by mother's socio-economic group (NS-SEC) (2000)

	Percentage who smoked before or during pregnancy	Percentage who smoked throughout pregnancy	Base: All stage 1 mothers*	Percentage who gave up before or during pregnancy	Base:: Stage 1 mothers who smoked before or during pregnancy
	%	%		%	
Higher occupations	22	7	1450	66	321
Intermediate occupations	29	13	986	56	284
Lower occupations	46	28	1356	38	619
Never worked	48	34	672	30	324
Unclassified	38	21	457	45	173
All mothers	**35**	**19**	**4921**	**45**	**1720**

*Excludes 200 mothers who did not supply sufficient information for classifying their smoking status.

Table 4.10

Smoking and pregnancy in England and Wales by mother's socio-economic group (NS-SEC) (2000)

	Percentage who smoked before or during pregnancy	Percentage who smoked throughout pregnancy	Base: All stage 1 mothers*	Percentage who gave up before or during pregnancy	Base:: Stage 1 mothers who smoked before or during pregnancy
	%	%		%	
Higher occupations	22	8	1534	65	340
Intermediate occupations	28	13	1049	55	298
Lower occupations	46	28	1437	39	666
Never worked	49	35	715	30	352
Unclassified	38	22	489	44	188
All mothers	**35**	**19**	**5224**	**45**	**1844**

*Excludes 216 mothers who did not supply sufficient information for classifying their smoking status.

Table 4.11

Smoking and pregnancy in Scotland by mother's socio-economic group (NS-SEC) (2000)

	Percentage who smoked before or during pregnancy	Percentage who smoked throughout pregnancy	Base: All stage 1 mothers*	Percentage who gave up before or during pregnancy	Base:: Stage 1 mothers who smoked before or during pregnancy
	%	%		%	
Higher occupations	21	10	691	53	143
Intermediate occupations	34	14	450	58	153
Lower occupations	48	33	593	31	283
Never worked	52	40	259	23	135
Unclassified	42	27	211	34	88
All mothers	**36**	**22**	**2206**	**39**	**802**

*Excludes 68 mothers who did not supply sufficient information for classifying their smoking status.

Table 4.12

Smoking and pregnancy in Northern Ireland by mother's socio-economic group (NS-SEC) (2000)

	Percentage who smoked before or during pregnancy	Percentage who smoked throughout pregnancy	Base: All stage 1 mothers*	Percentage who gave up before or during pregnancy	Base:: Stage 1 mothers who smoked before or during pregnancy
	%	%		%	
Higher occupations	20	11	475	46	96
Intermediate occupations	31	16	349	48	108
Lower occupations	45	29	485	35	219
Never worked	60	46	223	24	134
Unclassified	36	19	189	49	68
All mothers	**36**	**23**	**1722**	**38**	**625**

*Excludes 56 mothers who did not supply sufficient information for classifying their smoking status.

Tables 4.13 - 4.17 show the association between age of mother and smoking. Younger mothers were considerably more likely to smoke both before and during pregnancy in all countries. In the United Kingdom, around two thirds of teenage mothers smoked before they were pregnant and around four in ten continued to smoke throughout their pregnancy. This compares with under a quarter of older mothers over the age of 30 smoking before pregnancy and around one in eight continuing to smoke whilst pregnant.

Tables 4.13–4.17

Table 4.13
Smoking and pregnancy by mother's age (United Kingdom 2000)

	Percentage who smoked before or during pregnancy	Percentage who smoked throughout pregnancy	Base: All stage 1 mothers*	Percentage who gave up before or during pregnancy	Base:: Stage 1 mothers who smoked before or during pregnancy
	%	%		%	
Under 20	65	40	624	38	403
20 - 24	53	30	1583	43	841
25 - 29	36	20	2588	45	930
30 - 34	25	13	2806	48	697
35+	24	13	1502	45	355
All mothers**	**35**	**20**	**9126**	**44**	**3233**

*Excludes 366 mothers who did not supply sufficient information for classifying their smoking status.
** Includes some mothers for whom age not recorded

Table 4.14
Smoking and pregnancy in England by mother's age (2000)

	Percentage who smoked before or during pregnancy	Percentage who smoked throughout pregnancy	Base: All stage 1 mothers*	Percentage who gave up before or during pregnancy	Base:: Stage 1 mothers who smoked before or during pregnancy
	%	%		%	
Under 20	64	39	341	38	217
20 - 24	52	29	863	44	447
25 - 29	36	19	1391	45	497
30 - 34	25	12	1523	50	373
35+	23	12	808	48	187
All mothers**	**35**	**19**	**4940**	**45**	**1720**

*Excludes mothers who did not supply sufficient information for classifying their smoking status.
** Includes some mother for whom age not recorded

Table 4.29

Changes to drinking habits during pregnancy by whether woman was given advice on drinking (United Kingdom 2000)

	Given advice on drinking	Not given advice on drinking	All mothers who drank before pregnancy
	%	%	%
Gave up drinking during pregnancy	19	23	20
Drank less during pregnancy	67	59	65
No change/drank more	4	7	5
Base: Stage 1 mothers drinking before pregnancy	*6361*	*1906*	*8267*

5
Choice of feeding method

Summary

- Two-thirds (65%) of mothers in the United Kingdom said that they planned to breastfeed their baby, this figure ranging from 51% in Northern Ireland, to 60% in Scotland and 66% in England and Wales.

- First-time mothers were more likely to intend to breastfeed than mothers of later babies (70% compared to 60% in the UK). Among mothers of later babies, those who had breastfed their previous baby for at least 6 weeks were much more likely than mothers who had exclusively bottle fed their previous baby to plan to breastfeed (94% compared with 21%).

- The most common reason for choosing to breastfeed was that breastfeeding was best for the baby's health, followed by convenience. The most common reason for choosing to bottle-feed was that it allowed others to feed the baby, followed by a dislike of the "idea" of breastfeeding.

- Three-quarters (76%) of mothers were able to state a specific health benefit in breastfeeding. Knowledge about health benefits increased with age, educational level, and socio-economic group.

- There was a familial history in breastfeeding patterns, with mothers who thought that they had been breastfed themselves being more likely to plan to breastfeed their own baby (82%) compared with those who had been bottle-fed as a baby (56%). Mothers' feeding intentions were also associated with how their peer group fed their babies. Mothers whose friends mostly breastfed were more likely to breastfeed themselves (87%) than mothers whose friends mostly bottle-fed (51%).

- Mothers who attended ante-natal classes were more likely to intend to breastfeed (79%) than mothers who did not (57%). First-time mothers attending classes were particularly likely to intend to breastfeed if these classes included discussion about feeding (82% intending to breastfeed compared with 70% attending classes without such discussion).

- One in ten mothers who breastfed (9%) said that they felt pressured into this decision, rising to 12% of first-time mothers who breastfed. This pressure was mainly linked to midwives (76% of those feeling pressured).

This chapter covers how mothers planned to feed their baby, and the reasons that lay behind their choice. We also look at how social factors are associated with intentions to breastfeed, as well as contact with health professionals. Mothers' knowledge of the health benefits of breastfeeding is also explored.

5.1 Planned method of feeding

All mothers were asked how they had **intended** to feed their baby before the birth, regardless of how the baby was actually fed once born. Table 5.1 illustrates the feeding intentions of mothers prior to the birth of their baby, by birth order and survey year. In 2000, as in 1995, the majority of mothers said that they had planned before the birth how to feed their baby. Only 8% of all mothers, and 9% of mothers of first babies, had not decided on a feeding method.

The 2000 survey shows that the proportion of all mothers planning to breastfeed has remained unchanged since 1995, with 65% of mothers in the United Kingdom planning this. Mothers expecting their first baby in 2000 were more likely to plan to breastfeed than mothers having a later baby (70% compared to 60%). Compared with 1995, there was a small rise in the proportion of mothers with later babies planning to breastfeed (from 58% to 60%), although the rate among first babies remained unchanged.

Table 5.1

Table 5.1
Mother's intended method of feeding by birth order (1995 and 2000, United Kingdom)

	First births		Later births		All babies	
	1995 %	2000 %	1995 %	2000 %	1995 %	2000 %
Breast*	70	70	58	60	64	65
Not breast	22	21	37	33	30	27
Had not decided	8	9	5	6	6	8
Base(All Stage 1 mothers)	2,355	4,448	2,845	5,044	5,181	9,492

* Includes mothers who intended to combine breast and bottle feeding

Within individual countries, the percentage of mothers planning to breastfeed ranged from 66% in England and Wales to 60% in Scotland and 51% in Northern Ireland, this variation reflecting the differences between countries in the actual incidence of breastfeeding (see section 2.1). Also in line with changes in the incidence of breastfeeding, the proportion of mothers planning to breastfeed in Scotland and Northern Ireland had increased significantly since 1995. During this time period, intentions to breastfeed in Scotland rose from 54% to 60%, and in Northern Ireland from 44% to 51%.

Table 5.2

Table 5.2
Mother's intended method of feeding by country, 1995 and 2000

	England & Wales		Scotland		Northern Ireland		United Kingdom	
	1995 %	2000 %	1995 %	2000 %	1995 %	2000 %	1995 %	2000 %
Breast*	65	66	54	60	44	51	64	65
Not breast	29	26	38	31	48	40	30	27
Had not decided	6	7	8	9	8	9	6	8
Base (All Stage 1 mothers)	*4,598*	*5,441*	*1863*	*2,274*	*1476*	*1,778*	*5181*	*9,492*

* Includes mothers who intended to combine breast and bottle feeding

Figure 5.1 and Table 5.3 illustrate the effect that previous experience has on the intention of mothers of later babies to breastfeed. As in previous years, there was a strong correlation between previous experience of feeding and intentions regarding their latest baby. Mothers who had previously breastfed were more likely than others to intend to breastfeed their latest baby, and the longer they had breastfed the more likely this was to be the case. Six in ten mothers (60%) who had breastfed for less than six weeks, and 94% of mothers who had breastfed for longer than this planned to breastfeed their latest baby. This compares with a fifth (21%) of mothers who had not breastfed previous children, which is similar to the proportion (26%) who did actually switch to breast from bottle feeding for their later child (see section 2.2).

Table 5.3, Figure 5.1

Table 5.3
Mother's intended method of feeding by previous experience of breastfeeding (United Kingdom, 2000)

	Did not breastfeed	Breastfed for less than 6 weeks	Breastfed for 6 weeks or more	All later babies**
	%	%	%	%
Breast*	21	60	94	60
Not breast	69	30	3	33
Had not decided	9	10	2	6
Base (All Stage 1 mothers of later babies)	*1793*	*966*	*2068*	*5044*

* Includes mothers who intended to combine breast and bottle feeding
** Includes mothers where feeding history of previous baby unknown

Figure 5.1
Percentage of mothers planning to breastfeed by birth order and previous experience of breastfeeding

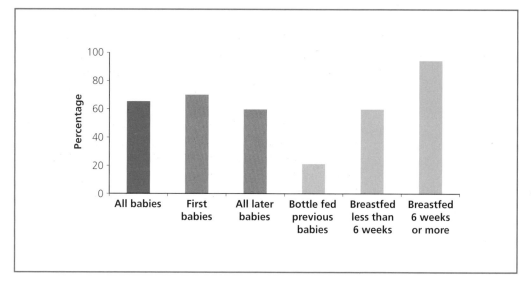

As found in previous surveys, almost all mothers (96%) carried out their stated intentions regarding feeding and this is illustrated in table 5.4. However, some caution should be placed on these high levels of correspondence as mothers asked retrospectively about their intentions may have forgotten, and/or rationalised, their behavioural intentions in the light of the method which they actually chose after the birth.

In general, mothers who planned to breastfeed were slightly more likely to have carried out their intentions compared with those who planned to bottle feed, although the correspondence between stated intentions and behaviour was almost universal in all cases.

Table 5.4

Table 5.4
Proportion of mothers who fed their baby in the way they had planned by method and country (2000)

	England & Wales	Scotland	Northern Ireland	United Kingdom
	Percentage feeding in way planned			
Breast	97	98	95	97
Not breast	94	95	94	94
All who planned	96	97	94	96
Bases (All Stage 1 mothers who had decided on method)				
Breast	*3,601*	*1,362*	*903*	*6,163*
Not breast	*1,410*	*696*	*712*	*2,564*
All who planned	*5,011*	*2,058*	*1,615*	*8,727*

5.2   Choice of feeding method

5.2.1   Reasons for choice

Mothers were asked their reasons behind their intended method of feeding. Table 5.5 illustrates the reasons given by those mothers who intended to breastfeed by birth order, and results are compared for 1995 and 2000. By far the most common response in 2000 was that breastfeeding was "best for the baby", this including all responses relating to the health of the baby including mentions of increased immunity to illness, nutrition, reduced risk of allergies as well as more general mentions of health benefits. This reason was cited by more mothers of first babies who intended to breastfeed (85%) than mothers of later babies (73%). The next most common reason, given by 37% of these mothers in 2000, was convenience; just under a quarter (23%) said that they chose breastfeeding as it could help to develop a closer bond between the mother and the baby, and a similar proportion (20%) cited the lack of cost as a factor.

Overall, responses given in 2000 were similar to those given in 1995.

Table 5.5

Table 5.5
Mother's reasons for planning to breastfeed by birth order (United Kingdom, 1995 & 2000)

	First births		Later births		All babies	
	1995 %	2000 %	1995 %	2000 %	1995 %	2000 %
Breastfeeding is best for baby	89	85	77	73	83	79
Breastfeeding is more convenient	36	34	37	40	37	37
Closer bond between mother and baby	21	23	19	23	20	23
Breastfeeding is cheaper/free	23	21	19	19	21	20
Breastfed previous baby (babies)	-	-	33	32	17	16
Breastfeeding is natural	14	14	10	11	12	12
Breastfeeding better for mother's health	13	13	10	11	12	12
Mother loses weight more easily**	n/a	13	n/a	9	n/a	11
Influenced by health professionals	3	4	2	2	3	3
Influenced by friends or relatives	2	4	1	1	2	3
History of allergies/illness in family*	n/a	3	n/a	3	n/a	3
No particular reason	0	3	0	4	0	3
Other reason	2	4	3	4	2	4
Base (Stage 1 mothers who planned to breastfeed)	*1,640*	*3,112*	*1,661*	*3,051*	*3,301*	*6,163*

* This code introduced in 2000
** In 1995, comments about mother losing weight were included in "Better for mother's health"
Percentages do not add to 100 as some mothers gave more than one reason

Table 5.6 displays the reasons why women of second or subsequent babies planned to breastfeed by whether mothers had breastfed previous children. This highlights the differences between mothers who were able to base their reasons on experience, against the small subsample of mothers who had had no prior experience and had decided to switch to breastfeeding after bottle-feeding previous children.

Women with previous experience of breastfeeding gave a more diverse set of reasons for wishing to breastfeed and placed much more emphasis on the practical benefits including convenience (42% compared with 23% of mothers with no experience of breastfeeding) and lack of cost (19% compared with 11%). They are also more likely to mention bonding between mother and child (24% compared with 9% of mothers with no previous experience), and inevitably a high proportion (37%) mention their experience of feeding previous children. Mothers with no previous experience mainly focussed on the health benefits for the baby (65%) and the convenience (23%) although a lower proportion mentioned both these aspects when compared to mothers with breastfeeding experience. Mothers with no previous experience of breastfeeding were more likely to give a non-specific response as to why they planned to breastfeed (13% compared with 3% of mothers with experience).

Table 5.6

Table 5.6

Mother's reasons for planning to breastfeed by previous experience of breastfeeding (United Kingdom, 2000)

	At least one breastfed	None breastfed
	%	%
Breastfeeding is best for baby	74	65
Breastfeeding is more convenient	42	23
Closer bond between mother and baby	24	9
Breastfeeding is cheaper/free	19	11
Breastfed previous baby (babies)*	37	-
Breastfeeding is natural	11	5
Breastfeeding is better for mother's health	12	9
Mother loses weight more easily**	10	6
Influenced by health professionals	2	3
Influenced by friends or relatives	1	2
History of allergies/illness in family*	3	3
No particular reason	3	13
Other reason	3	8
Base (Stage 1 mothers with more than one child who planned to breastfeed)	2663	316

Table 5.7 illustrates the most common reasons for intending to use infant formula rather than breastfeed, and data is shown by birth order for the last two survey years. In 2000, the main responses given by women for planning to bottle-feed are the flexibility of other people being able to feed baby (25%), simply not liking the "idea" of breastfeeding (19%), and because of previous experience of bottle-feeding (15%).

First-time mothers were more likely than mothers of later babies to object to the "idea" of breastfeeding (27% compared with 15%). One in six mothers of later babies (16%) mentioned having breastfed a previous baby and being put off by the experience.

Compared with 1995, mothers in 2000 who had planned to bottle-feed were less likely to mention the flexibility aspect of others feeding the baby (25% compared with 36% in 1995) and being put off by the idea of breastfeeding (19% compared with 27%).

Table 5.7

Table 5.7
Mother's reasons for planning to bottle feed by birth order (United Kingdom, 1995 & 2000)

	First births		Later births		All babies	
	1995 %	**2000** %	**1995** %	**2000** %	**1995** %	**2000** %
Other people can feed baby	46	29	32	22	36	25
Did not like the idea of breastfeeding	34	27	23	15	27	19
Bottle-fed previous children*	}-	-	}44	23	}30	15
Breastfed previous children and didn't get on with it*		-		16		10
Can see how much the baby has had	7	7	5	4	6	5
Would be embarrassed to breastfeed	11	4	4	4	7	4
Expecting to return to work soon	12	7	3	2	6	4
Bottle feeding is less tiring	2	2	6	2	4	2
Medical reasons for not breastfeeding	3	2	4	4	4	4
No particular reason	2	5	1	3	1	4
Other reason	6	6	5	5	6	5
Base (Stage 1 mothers who planned to bottlefeed)	*513*	*921*	*1,044*	*1,642*	*1,557*	*2,563*

* In 1995, these two codes were combined
Percentages do not add to 100 as some mothers gave more than one reason

A fifth (19%) of mothers planning to bottle-feed had breastfed a previous baby in the past. Nearly half (46%) of this subgroup cited being put off by past experience of breastfeeding as a reason for choosing bottle-feeding this time round.

5.3 Awareness of health benefits of breastfeeding

For the first time, the 2000 survey explored mothers' awareness of the health benefits in breastfeeding. The majority of mothers (86%) said that were aware of health benefits in breastfeeding and this was broadly the same across all countries. However, when asked to state what they thought these benefits were, 12% of this subgroup did not give an answer. It could be argued that those mothers who were unable to give an answer to this question were not truly knowledgeable, and if these mothers are omitted from analysis the proportion who are aware of health benefits reduces to 76%.

Table 5.8 displays the proportion who say that they were aware of the health benefits of breastfeeding in total, together with the adjusted proportion (i.e. those aware and able to give a substantiating reason). The commentary which follows refers to the adjusted proportion as this is considered to be a more accurate gauge of mothers' knowledge.

By country, there is little variation in the proportion of mothers aware and able to give a reason. However, there are clear variations by demographic subgroups. Knowledge about health benefits increases with age, with 80% of mothers aged at least 30 claiming to be aware compared with 57% of teenage mothers. There is also a strong gradient by socio-economic group with 89% of mothers in higher occupations aware reducing to 73% of mothers in lower occupations and 54% of those who have never worked.

White women and those of mixed or other ethnic origins were more knowledgeable according to this measure with around three-quarters being aware compared with three in five mothers from Black and Asian ethnic groups. This differential is interesting given that Asian and Black women are more likely to initiate breastfeeding than white women (see section 2.1). Thus the data would suggest that the increased propensity of mothers from Asian and Black ethnic backgrounds to breastfeed is not driven by a better knowledge of the beneficial effects of breastfeeding, but is perhaps linked to a more general cultural influence.

We also looked at mother's knowledge of the health benefits of breastfeeding by how mothers planned to feed, and experience of feeding any previous children. Mothers planning to breastfeed were much more likely to be aware of the benefits (83%) compared with those who planned to bottle-feed (60%). And mothers who had breastfed before were much more likely to show an awareness (81%) compared with those who had had previous children but had never breastfed (61%)

Table 5.8

Mothers who said that they were aware of health benefits were asked what these were. Answers were collected as an open response and later coded into a codeframe. Answers given by more than 5% of the subset of mothers who were aware of health benefits are shown in table 5.9

The most commonly cited health benefit was the increased immunity against illness offered to babies through breastmilk. Three quarters of mothers in the United Kingdom aware of health benefits mentioned this. Other benefits for the baby mentioned by at least a fifth of this subset of mothers were breastmilk being more nutritious (37%), reduced likelihood of asthma, eczema or other allergies (23%), and reduced likelihood of colic/wind (20%). Some mothers also mentioned benefits for the mother including helping her uterus to contract (23%) and a reduction in the risk of breast or ovarian cancer (19%).

Mothers in Scotland who showed an awareness of health benefits were less likely than mothers in other countries to mention nutrition (24% compared with 38% in England & Wales and 36% in Northern Ireland) but were more likely to mention reduced risk of allergies (32% compared with 23% and 25%) and reduced risk of cancer for mothers (31% compared with 18% and 19%).

Table 5.9

Table 5.8
Proportion of mothers who say they are aware of health benefits by country, mother's age, age completed full-time education, mother's socio-economic group (NS-SEC), ethnicity, how planned to feed baby and whether previous children breastfed (United Kingdom, 2000)

	Proportion aware of health benefits	Proportion aware of health benefits and able to give reason	Base
All Stage 1 mothers*	86	76	9492
Country			
England & Wales	85	76	5441
Scotland	88	77	2274
Northern Ireland	86	74	1778
Mother's age			
Under 20	64	57	657
20-24	78	69	1670
25-29	88	77	2703
30+	90	80	4428
Mother's socio-economic group (NS-SEC)			
Higher occupations	96	89	2791
Intermediate occupations	91	81	1906
Lower occupations	83	73	2619
Never worked	65	54	1276
Unclassified	79	61	901
Ethnicity			
White	87	77	8609
Asian	68	60	275
Black	79	60	184
Mixed	81	76	93
Other	74	62	66
How planned to feed baby			
Planned to breastfeed	91	83	6162
Planned to bottle-feed	73	60	2564
Did not plan feeding method	82	70	713
Whether previous children breastfed			
Yes, previous child breastfed	91	81	3336
No, none breastfed	75	61	1577
First-time mother (no previous children)	85	77	4448

* Includes some mothers for whom there are missing values on some of the variables tabulated

Table 5.11

Proportion of mothers who planned to breastfeed their baby by how most of her friends fed their babies and by country, 2000

	England & Wales	Scotland	Northern Ireland	United Kingdom	England & Wales	Scotland	Northern Ireland	United Kingdom
	Percentage who planned to breastfeed				Bases			
Most breastfed	87	85	81	87	1,217	489	209	2,063
Half breast/half not breast	70	63	56	69	1,263	497	342	2,174
Most did not breastfeed	53	47	43	51	2,061	970	1,039	3,733
Don't know other mothers	67	55	[18]	65	919	56	[35]	1010
All Stage 1 mothers	**66**	60	**51**	**65**	**5,438**	**2,273**	**1,777**	**9,492**

* Bases do not sum to total due to missing data on how friends fed babies (including "don't know how other mothers feed babies")

Figure 5.3

Proportion of mothers who planned to breastfeed their baby by how most of her friends feed babies

Base: All Stage 1 mothers

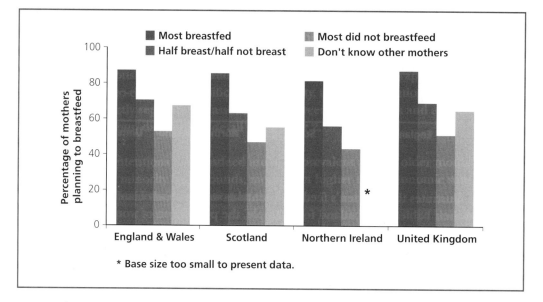

* Base size too small to present data.

5.5 Contact with health professionals

As shown in previous surveys, almost all mothers (98%) had had some antenatal check-ups during pregnancy. Mothers were asked whether anyone had asked about their feeding intentions during these check-ups and whether anyone had discussed feeding with them. Given that some of these discussions may have taken place up to a year before the survey questionnaire was completed some caution should be placed on the results due to memory recall error.

Table 5.12 shows that seven in ten mothers (68%) in the United Kingdom recalled discussing feeding at their ante-natal check-ups, this figure being higher for mothers expecting their first baby (70%) than for those who already had children (65%). By country, mothers in Scotland were the most likely to have discussed feeding during ante-natal check-ups (79%), while mothers in England and Wales were the least likely (66%).

Around one in six mothers (17% in the United Kingdom) recalled being asked about their feeding intentions but did not recall any discussion about this. The proportion of mothers who did not remember discussing any aspect of feeding was 13% in the United Kingdom. Mothers in England and Wales were more likely than mothers in other countries to have not discussed any aspect of feeding (15% compared with 6% in Scotland and 10% in Northern Ireland).

Table 5.12

Table 5.12
Whether mother was asked about plans or discussed feeding at antenatal check-ups
by birth order and country, 2000

	England & Wales			Scotland			Northern Ireland			United Kingdom		
	First births %	Later births %	All %	First births %	Later births %	All %	First births %	Later births %	All %	First births %	Later births %	All %
Had discussion about feeding	69	64	66	82	76	79	78	71	74	70	65	68
No discussion but asked about plans	15	20	17	12	17	14	12	17	15	15	19	17
No discussion and not asked about plans	14	14	15	5	6	6	9	11	10	13	15	13
All who had antenatal check-ups	98	98	98	99	99	99	99	99	99	98	99	98
Base (All Stage 1 mothers)	2560	2881	5441	1115	1159	2274	729	1049	1778	4,448	5,044	9492

Table 5.13 shows the proportion of mothers discussing feeding at ante-natal check-ups by survey year. Between 1995 and 2000 there was an increase in the proportion of mothers who had discussed feeding during antenatal checks from 58% to 68%. This increase was evident for both first births (from 64% to 70%) and for later births (from 53% to 65%).

Table 5.13

Table 5.13
Whether mother was asked about plans or discussed feeding at antenatal check-ups by birth order (United Kingdom 1995 and 2000)

	First births		Later births		All babies	
	1995 **%**	**2000** **%**	**1995** **%**	**2000** **%**	**1995** **%**	**2000** **%**
Had discussion about feeding	64	70	53	65	58	68
No discussion but asked about plans	23	15	33	19	29	17
No discussion and not asked about plans	12	13	13	15	12	13
All who had antenatal check-ups	99	98	99	98	99	98
Base (All Stage 1 mothers)	*2332*	*4448*	*2840*	*5044*	*5172*	*9492*

As discussed in the previous chapter, mothers were asked if they had gone to classes to prepare for having their baby and whether the classes had included any talks or discussions about feeding. Table 5.14 illustrates that women expecting their first child were more likely than mothers of later babies to have been to antenatal classes and, as most classes included talks or discussions about feeding, they were also more likely to have attended talks on feeding. In the United Kingdom, just over half (52%) of mothers of first babies and less than one in ten (8%) of mothers of later babies had been to classes that included talks on feeding.

Compared with the other countries, mothers in Scotland were more likely to attend antenatal classes, and they were also more likely to have discussed feeding. This difference is seen for both first and later births.

Table 5.14

Table 5.14
Whether mother went to classes to prepare for having the baby and whether classes included talks or discussions about feeding by country, 2000

	England & Wales			Scotland			Northern Ireland			United Kingdom		
	First births %	Later births %	All %	First births %	Later births %	All %	First births %	Later births %	All %	First births %	Later births %	All %
Went to classes	64	11	36	74	20	46	65	9	32	64	11	36
Went to classes with talks on feeding	51	8	28	59	12	35	53	6	25	52	8	28
Base (All Stage 1 mothers)	*2560*	*2881*	*5441*	*1115*	*1159*	*2274*	*729*	*1049*	*1778*	*4,448*	*5,044*	*9492*

Table 5.15 compares the proportions of mothers who intended to breastfeed according to whether they had discussed feeding at antenatal check-ups or classes. As in 1995,

discussion of feeding at antenatal check-ups was not found to be associated with the intention to breastfeed, and this was the case for both first and later births.

Attendance at antenatal classes, however, shows a stronger association with feeding intentions and a positive relationship between attendance at classes and the intention to breastfeed is clear. Mothers who had not attended classes were less likely than others to plan to breastfeed (57%). There also appears to be a small effect from attending classes which specifically included discussion about feeding. Four-fifths (81%) of mothers attending classes which included this intended to breastfeed compared with 71% of mothers who attended classes but without such discussion. This differential was concentrated solely within the first-time mothers; mothers expecting later babies were as likely to intend to breastfeed regardless of whether their classes included this subject matter.

Table 5.15

Table 5.15
Proportion of mothers intending to breastfeed by whether discussed feeding at antenatal check-ups or whether went to classes with talks about feeding, by birth order (United Kingdom, 2000)

	First births	Later births	All	First birth	Later birth	All
	Percentage to be breastfed			*Bases*		
Antenatal check-ups						
Discussed feeding at antenatal check-ups	70	60	65	*3,129*	*3,287*	*6,417*
Did not discuss or did not have check-up	69	60	64	*1,265*	*1,695*	*2,960*
Antenatal classes						
Went to classes with talks or discussion about feeding	82	77	81	*2,306*	*394*	*2,699*
Went to classes, no talks on feeding	70	76	71	*551*	*182*	*732*
Did not go to classes	52	58	57	*1,555*	*4,432*	*5,986*
*All Stage 1 mothers**	*70*	*60*	*65*	*4,448*	*5,044*	*9,492*

* Bases do not sum to total as not all mothers answered the questions on antenatal care.

For the first time in 2000, the issue of whether or not the mother ever felt pressured into making her decision on how to feed her baby was explored in more depth. Table 5.16 illustrates that, overall, nine in ten mothers (90%) reported that they did not feel pressurised into their choice of feeding method. Of those mothers who did feel pressured into making a decision, the large majority felt pressured into breast (8%) as opposed to bottle-feeding (1%). These proportions were broadly the same across all countries. There a small but significant difference in the proportion of first-time mothers feeling pressured into breastfeeding (10%) when compared to mothers of later babies (6%).

Table 5.16

Table 5.16

Proportion of mothers who felt pressured into making decision on how to feed baby by country and birth order, 2000

	England & Wales			Scotland			Northern Ireland			United Kingdom		
	First births %	Later births %	All %	First births %	Later births %	All %	First births %	Later births %	All %	First births %	Later births %	All %
Felt pressured into breastfeeding	10	6	8	7	5	6	9	5	7	10	6	8
Felt pressured into bottle feeding	2	1	2	1	1	1	1	1	1	2	1	1
Did not feel pressured into either	86	92	89	91	93	92	89	93	91	87	92	90
Base (All Stage 1 mothers)	*2560*	*2881*	*5441*	*1115*	*1159*	*2274*	*729*	*1049*	*1778*	*4,448*	*5,044*	*9492*

The above table illustrates the proportion who felt pressured into making particular feeding decisions based on **all** mothers. Table 5.17 shows, by birth order within country, the proportion of all mothers **breastfeeding at birth** who felt pressured into making this decision. This shows that 12% of first-time mothers in the United Kingdom who chose to breastfeed felt some pressure to do this, this figure being slightly lower in Scotland (9%).

Table 5.17

Table 5.17

Proportion of mothers breastfeeding at birth who felt pressured into breastfeeding by country and birth order, 2000

	England & Wales			Scotland			Northern Ireland			United Kingdom		
	First births %	Later births %	All %	First births %	Later births %	All %	First births %	Later births %	All %	First births %	Later births %	All %
Felt pressured into breastfeeding	12	7	10	9	7	8	12	7	9	12	7	9
Base (All Stage 1 mothers who breastfed initially)	*1932*	*1905*	*3837*	*747*	*684*	*1431*	*430*	*533*	*963*	*3296*	*3266*	*6562*

It is interesting to compare the duration of breastfeeding for those mothers who felt some pressure to do so with the duration for all breastfeeding mothers. Table 5.18 shows that those mothers who felt under pressure were much more likely than average to give up breastfeeding within the first few weeks. Over a third (36%) gave up within the first two weeks, compared with 21% of all breastfeeding mothers. By 4 months, a quarter of breastfeeding mothers who felt pressured were still breastfeeding, compared with 44% of all breastfeeding mothers.

Table 5.18

Table 5.18
Duration of breastfeeding for those who breastfed initially by whether felt pressured into breastfeeding (United Kingdom, 2000)

	Breastfeeding mothers who felt pressured	All breastfeeding mothers
	%	%
Birth	100	100
1 week	72	84
2 weeks	64	79
6 weeks	44	64
4 months (17 weeks)	26	44
6 months (26 weeks)	20	34
9 months (39 weeks)	11	19
Base (Stage 3 mothers who breastfed initially)	*428*	*5023*

Mothers who did feel under some pressure to feed in a particular way were asked to indicate who had made them feel this way. The figures are shown in Table 5.19 individually for mothers who felt pressured into breast and bottle feeding. The large majority of mothers feeling pressured into breastfeeding felt this pressure from midwives (76%); a quarter (25%) felt under pressure from health visitors and 20% from friends. For the small subset of mothers who felt under pressure to bottle-feed this push was much less likely to come from health professional sources. Just over a third (37%) of bottle-feeding mothers under pressure mentioned midwives, and only 12% mentioned the health visitor. However, they were more likely than breastfeeding mothers to cite their own mother as a source of pressure (25% compared with 11% of breastfeeding mothers).

Table 5.19

Table 5.19
Who made mothers feel pressured into breastfeeding and bottle feeding (United Kingdom, 2000)

	Mothers feeling pressured into breastfeeding	Mothers feeling pressured into bottle feeding
	%	%
Midwife	76	37
Health visitor	25	12
Friends/other mothers	20	20
Partner	16	17
Doctor/GP	16	12
Nurse	15	11
Mother	11	25
Voluntary organisation (e.g. National Childbirth Trust)	7	-
Grandmother	3	5
Base (All Stage 1 mothers feeling pushed into feeding method)	*734*	*138*

6

The birth & post-natal care

Summary

- The type of analgesic given to mothers during labour had an effect on their likelihood to breastfeed, with mothers who were given a general anaesthetic being less likely to start breastfeeding (62%) than mothers who had an epidural (71%) or no analgesic at all (72%).

- Mothers who experienced a delay before they first fed their baby were more likely to have given up breastfeeding in the first two weeks than were mothers who breastfed their baby immediately.

- If the baby was given formula milk in hospital, it is a strong indicator that the mother will not continue breastfeeding after leaving hospital. Two fifths (40%) of breastfeeding mothers whose babies had been given a bottle while in hospital had stopped breastfeeding within two weeks, compared with one in eight breastfeeding mothers (13%) whose babies had not been given a bottle.

- 32% of breastfeeding mothers experienced problems feeding their baby in hospital. Although the group is small, mothers who did not receive help for these problems were more likely to have given up breastfeeding within the first two weeks (47%) than those who received help (29%). A similar proportion of breastfeeding mothers (35%) experienced feeding problems once they had left hospital and, again, those who did not receive help for these problems were more likely to have given up breastfeeding by two weeks (32%) than those who had received help (15%).

- 13% of bottle-feeding mothers experienced feeding problems in hospital and 12% experienced problems after they left. Compared with breastfeeding mothers who had problems, bottle-feeding mothers were more likely to cite difficulties relating to the health of the baby including vomiting and colic.

- The support of relatives and friends had a strong influence on the likelihood of breastfeeding mothers to continue breastfeeding beyond the first two weeks. Breastfeeding mothers who were themselves bottle fed were more likely to give up (24%) than those who had been breastfed themselves (15%). Similarly, breastfeeding mothers whose friends mostly bottle fed were more likely to have given up by two weeks (30%) than those whose friends mostly breastfed (10%).

- 80% of mothers followed the advice related to avoiding cot death and placed their baby to sleep on his or her back.

Reasons for giving up breastfeeding

Mothers who gave up breastfeeding were asked their reasons for doing so. The main reasons given by mothers who gave up within the first 2 weeks were that their baby did not suck or rejected the breast (31%), that they had insufficient milk (29%), and that they had painful breasts (27%).

Reasons given by mothers who gave up in the first week varied slightly from those given by mothers who gave up in the second week. Those who gave up in the first week were most likely to cite the fact that their baby would not suck or rejected the breast (35% compared with 19% of those giving up in the second week), whereas the reason most mentioned by those giving up in the second week was an insufficiency of milk (41% compared with 26% of those giving up in the first week). Other common reasons at this stage included painful breasts and the fact that breastfeeding took too long. The latter was more likely to be considered a problem in the second than in the first week (17% compared with 11%).

The importance of other reasons also differed according to whether mothers had given up in the first or second week after the birth. Mothers who gave up in the first few days were more likely to say that they did not like breastfeeding; those who continued breastfeeding for between one and two weeks were more likely to cite domestic reasons.

Table 6.8

Table 6.8
Reasons given by mothers for stopping breastfeeding within one or two weeks
(1995 GB, 2000 UK)*

| | Baby's age when breastfeeding ceased | | | |
| | less than 1 week | | 1 week but less than 2 weeks | |
	1995	2000	1995	2000
Insufficient milk	32	26	44	41
Painful breasts or nipples	28	27	36	29
Baby would not suck / rejected breast	29	35	20	19
Breastfeeding took too long/ was tiring	11	11	16	17
Mother was ill	11	8	16	12
Did not like breastfeeding	10	8	5	4
Domestic reasons	6	4	10	8
Baby was ill	7	5	4	10
Difficult to judge how much baby drunk	4	3	2	2
Baby could not be fed by others	3	1	1	2
Other reasons	14	14	16	16
Base (Stage 1 breastfeeding mothers who gave up within first 2 weeks)	*480*	*1069*	*164*	*318*

* Note that 1995 data based on GB, 2000 data based on UK

There were also differences in reasons given for stopping breastfeeding in the first two weeks between first-time and more experienced mothers. The main reason given by first-time mothers giving up breastfeeding in the first two weeks was that the baby would not suck or rejected the breast (38% of these mothers mentioned this, compared with 23% of more experienced mothers). For both groups of mothers this was especially an issue in the first week of the baby's life. However, by the second week, whereas only 6% of more experienced mothers gave up breastfeeding because of their baby rejecting the breast, this was still the cause of stopping breastfeeding for three in ten first-time mothers (30%).

Mothers of second or later babies were more likely to mention painful breasts or nipples as a reason for giving up in the first two weeks (31% compared with 24% first time mothers). They were also more likely to cite the fact that breastfeeding took a long time and was tiring (15%, 10% of first time mothers) and domestic reasons (10%, compared with less than 1% of first-time mothers), issues that could be caused or exacerbated by the presence of other children.

Table 6.9

Table 6.9
Reasons given by mothers for stopping breastfeeding within 1 or 2 weeks, first births vs. later births (United Kingdom 2000)

| | Baby's age when breastfeeding ceased | | | | | |
| | less than 1 week | | 1 week but less than 2 weeks | | Up to 2 weeks | |
	First births %	Later births %	First births %	Later births %	First births %	Later births %
Insufficient milk	26	26	45	34	30	28
Painful breasts or nipples	23	31	28	31	24	31
Baby would not suck / rejected breast	40	28	30	6	38	23
Breastfeeding took too long/ was tiring	9	14	16	17	10	15
Mother was ill	9	7	11	12	10	8
Did not like breastfeeding	9	6	2	6	7	6
Domestic reasons	*	8	0	19	*	10
Baby was ill	7	4	12	7	8	4
Difficult to judge how much baby drunk	4	2	1	3	3	2
Baby could not be fed by others	2	*	2	1	2	*
Mother had inverted nipples	2	2	-	-	2	2
Embarrassment	1	3	-	1	1	2
Returning to work	1	*	-	-	1	*
Other reasons	13	7	16	14	14	9
Base						
(Stage 1 breastfeeding mothers who gave up within first 2 weeks)	*617*	*452*	*179*	*140*	*796*	*592*

Delays in starting breastfeeding

Between 1995 and 2000 there was an increase in the proportion of mothers who began breastfeeding within one hour of giving birth. The proportion rose from 68% in 1995 to 72% in 2000.

Table 6.10

Table 6.10

Length of time before baby was first put to the breast (1990, 1995 Great Britain, 2000 United Kingdom)*

	1990 %	1995 %	2000 %
Immediately / within a few minutes	26	25	28
Within an hour	37	43	44
More than 1 hour, up to 4 hours later	18	17	14
More than 4 hours, up to 12 hours later	10	8	5
More than 12 hours later	10	8	7
Base *(Stage 1 breast feeding mothers who had hospital birth)*	*3,395*	*3,337*	*6,354*

* Note that 1990 and 1995 data based on GB, 2000 data based on UK

The duration of breastfeeding continued to show a relationship with the length of time before the baby is put to the breast. Delays in first feeds were associated with an increasing likelihood of stopping breastfeeding in the first two weeks. In 2000, 16% of mothers who breastfed immediately had given up by the end of the second week, compared with 26% of those who, for one reason or another, had not put their baby to the breast for more than an hour after birth.

However, although mothers were more likely to begin breastfeeding within one hour of giving birth in 2000 than in 1995, there was also an increase in the proportion of these mothers giving up breastfeeding within two weeks (19% in 2000 compared with 15% in 1995).

Table 6.11

Table 6.11

Proportion of mothers who had stopped breastfeeding within two weeks by the length of time taken to first put baby to breast. (1990, 1995 GB, 2000 UK)**

	1990	1995	2000	1990	1995	2000`
	Percentage stopping breastfeeding within 2 weeks				*Bases*	
Immediately	12	14	16	*843*	*804*	*1,790*
Within an hour	18	16	21	*1,196*	*1,381*	*2,796*
More than 1, up to 4 hours later	25	26	24	*593*	*564*	*862*
More than 4 hours, up to 12 hours later	24	26	30	*328*	*249*	*331*
More than 12 hours later	32	30	27	*314*	*252*	*467*
Stage 1 breastfeeding mothers who had hospital birth	*19*	*19*	*21*	*3,395*	*3,337*	*6,354*

*Includes some cases where the time until baby was put to breast was not known
** Note that 1990 and 1995 data based on GB, 2000 data based on UK

The prevalence of breastfeeding at 2 weeks did not show a statistically significant relationship with whether the baby was in special care, whether it had a low birthweight or whether there was a delay before the mother held her baby.

Contact between mother and baby in hospital

Babies kept by the mother's side at all times makes it easier for the mother to breastfeed on demand. The practice of placing some newborn babies in a nursery had continued to decline so that, by 2000, 79% of mothers had their baby with them continuously in hospital, compared to 74% in 1995 and 63% in 1990. A further 7% always fed their baby even though they were sometimes separated and a similar proportion were in special care most of the time. There was a further decrease in the proportion of babies who were sometimes fed by a nurse or midwife between 1995 and 2000, from 8% to 6%.

Table 6.12

Table 6.12
Contact between breastfeeding mothers and babies while in hospital (1990, 1995 GB, 2000 UK)*

	1990 %	1995 %	2000 %
Mother and baby together continuously	63	74	79
Baby away sometimes:			
Mother always fed baby	15	9	7
Nurses sometimes fed baby	16	8	6
Baby in incubator or special care most of the time (more than 1 day)	7	9	8
Base			
(Stage 1 breastfeeding mothers who had a hospital birth)	*3,392*	*3,243*	*6,354*

* Note that 1990 and 1995 data based on GB, 2000 data based on UK

Giving bottles to breastfed babies

Previous surveys have showed a strong association between giving bottles of formula milk to breastfed babies in hospital and the likelihood of the mother stopping breastfeeding in the early weeks. Between 1995 and 2000 there was a fall in the proportion of breastfed babies who were given bottles in hospital, from 36% to 28%. This followed on from decreases from 1985 to 1990 and from 1990 to 2000.

Table 6.13, Figure 6.1

Table 6.13
Frequency with which bottles of formula milk were given to breastfed babies in hospital (1990, 1995 GB, 2000 UK)*

	1990 %		1995 %		2000 %	
No bottles given	54		61		69	
Bottles given once or twice only	23		20		15	
Bottles given during the night	6		4		3	
Bottles given at every feed	9	45	7	36	7	28
Bottles given, other arrangements	5		5		3	
Bottles given, mother not sure how often	2		-		1	
Mother uncertain whether bottles given	1		3		*	
Base						
(Stage 1 breastfeeding mothers who had hospital birth)	*3,392*		*3,243*		*6,354*	

* Note that 1990 and 1995 data based on GB, 2000 data based on UK

Figure 6.1
Frequency with which bottles of formula milk were given to breastfed babies in hospital (1990, 1995 GB, 2000 UK).

Breast feeding mothers who had a hospital birth

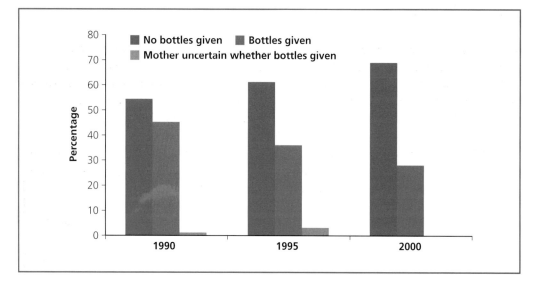

Breastfeeding mothers whose babies were given bottles were still more likely to stop breastfeeding in the first two weeks than were other mothers. Two fifths (40%) of breastfeeding mothers whose babies had been given a bottle while in hospital had stopped breastfeeding at this stage compared with 13% of breastfeeding mothers whose babies had not been given a bottle. Three fifths of mothers (60%) whose babies had been given a bottle at most feeds while in hospital had given up by two weeks. However, this measurement might reflect the proportion of mothers who were already having difficulties breastfeeding rather than the use of formula milk having an effect on their behaviour.

Table 6.14

Table 6.14
Proportion of mothers who had stopped breastfeeding within two weeks by frequency with which bottles of milk had been given in hospital (1990, 1995 GB, 2000 UK)*

	1990	1995	2000	1990	1995	2000`
Frequency of giving bottles of milk in hospital	*Percentage who had given up breastfeeding within 2 weeks*				*Bases*	
No bottles given	9	11	13	1,759	1,983	4,368
Bottles given occasionally or at night	23	27	33	939	746	1,136
Bottle given at most feeds	56	58	60	295	229	444
All babies who received a bottle while being breastfed	32	34	40	1,438	1,142	1,800
All Stage 1 breastfed babies born in hospital**	**20**	**20**	**21**	**3,392**	**2,243**	**6,354**

* Note that 1990 and 1995 data based on GB, 2000 data based on UK
** Includes some babies for whom whether bottles given not known

6.3 Problems feeding the baby and the role of health professionals

In 2000, 87% of mothers of first babies were given help, usually by a midwife or a nurse, the first time that they breastfed their baby. Mothers of second or later babies were understandably much less likely to receive advice at this stage. Although being shown how to breastfeed did not significantly affect the chances of the mother continuing to breastfeed, 94% of mothers said that they found the advice helpful.

Three fifths (62%) of mothers of first babies who did not receive help (8% of mothers of first babies) would have liked to have done so and a similar proportion (8%) of mothers of second or later babies would have liked to receive advice.

Table 6.15

Table 6.15

Proportion of breastfeeding mothers who received help or advice the first time they breastfed (United Kingdom 2000)

.

	Birth order		
	First births %	**Later births** %	**All babies** %
Received advice	87	48	67
Did not receive advice	13	51	32
Of which ... would have liked advice	8	8	8
... did not want advice	4	41	23
Base *(Stage 1 breast feeding mothers)*	*3,295*	*3,265*	*6,561*

Problems feeding the baby in hospital

While in hospital, 32% of breastfeeding mothers experienced problems feeding their baby, slightly fewer than in 1995, when 35% of breastfeeding mothers experienced problems. Not surprisingly, mothers of first babies were more likely to report problems (44%) than mothers of second or later babies (21%). As in previous surveys, the most common problems were that the baby would not suck or latch on to the breast (53% of mothers who experienced problems with breastfeeding) or that the mother had sore or cracked nipples (19% of mothers who experienced problems with breastfeeding). A further one in seven mothers who experienced problems (14%) mentioned that the baby appeared to be hungry or that they didn't have enough milk.

Table 6.16, 6.17

Table 6.16

Feeding problems experienced by breastfeeding mothers while in hospital (1990, 1995 GB, 2000 UK)*

	First births			Later births			All babies		
	1990 %	**1995** %	**2000** %	**1990** %	**1995** %	**2000** %	**1990** %	**1995** %	**2000** %
Had problems	47	46	44	25	24	21	36	35	32
Did not have problems	53	54	56	75	76	79	64	65	67
Base *(Stage 1* *breastfeeding mothers* *who had hospital birth)*	*1,657*	*1,638*	*3,247*	*1,681*	*1,583*	*3,107*	*3,338*	*3,243*	*6,354*

* Note that 1995 data based on GB, 2000 data based on UK

Table 6.17

Feeding problems experienced by breastfeeding mothers while in hospital or after leaving hospital, by birth order (United Kingdom 2000)

	Problems in hospital			Problems after leaving hospital		
	First birth	Later birth	All breastfed babies	First birth	Later birth	All breastfed babies
	Percentage having problem					
Baby would not suck/ not latching on	57	42	53	25	22	24
Mother had sore or cracked nipples	18	20	19	38	43	40
Baby unsatisfied/ insufficient milk	14	13	14	32	31	32
Baby was ill (in special care or fed by tube)	7	12	9	1	*	1
Baby falling asleep/ slow feeding/ not gaining weight	9	8	9	13	10	12
Lack of support/ advice from midwife/ nurse/ hospital	6	3	5	3	2	2
Mother too tired / ill	5	5	5	6	6	6
Mother found breastfeeding uncomfortable	2	2	2	3	2	2
Baby vomiting	1	3	2	3	4	3
Baby had colic/wind	1	*	1	6	8	7
Baby didn't like milk	*	*	*	*	1	1
Baby constipated	-	-	-	1	1	1
Other problems affecting mother	3	3	3	6	5	5
Other problems with baby	10	10	10	7	7	7
Base *(Stage 1 breastfeeding mothers* *who had feeding problems)*	*1,413*	*636*	*2,049*	*1,091*	*836*	*1,927*

One in eight mothers bottle-feeding in hospital (13%) said that they had experienced feeding problems. Compared with breastfeeding mothers, problems experienced by bottle-feeding mothers in hospital were more likely to be related to the health of the baby including baby being ill (20% compared with 9% of breastfeeding mothers reporting problems), baby vomiting (22% compared with 2%) and colic (4% compared with 1%). One in ten mothers with problems in hospital (11%) said that this because their baby wouldn't feed from a bottle.

Table 6.18

Table 6.18

Feeding problems experienced by mothers while in hospital or after leaving hospital, by feeding method at the time (United Kingdom 2000)

	Problems in hospital			Problems after leaving hospital		
	Breastfed	Not Breastfed	All babies	Breasted	Not breastfed	All babies
	Percentage having problem					
Any problem	32	13	26	35	12	26
Base:						
All mothers having hospital birth	2869	6353	9222	5557	3588	9145
Baby would not suck/ not latching on	53	13	46	24	2	20
Mother had sore or cracked nipples	19	*	16	40	-	33
Baby unsatisfied/ insufficient milk	14	4	12	32	32	32
Baby was ill (in special care or fed by tube)	9	20	10	1	1	1
Baby falling asleep/ slow feeding/ not gaining weight	9	12	9	12	10	11
Baby vomiting	2	22	5	3	22	7
Mother too tired / ill	5	3	5	6	1	5
Lack of support/ advice from midwife/ nurse/ hospital	5	1	4	2	1	2
Baby wouldn't feed from bottle	1	11	3	1	1	1
Mother found breastfeeding uncomfortable	2	-	2	2	-	2
Baby didn't like milk	*	1	1	1	1	1
Baby had colic/wind	1	4	1	7	27	11
Baby constipated	-	-	-	1	9	2
Other problems affecting mother	3	2	3	5	1	4
Other problems with baby	10	21	12	7	15	8
Base (Stage 1 mothers who had feeding problems)	2,049	358	2426	1,927	414	2340

The majority of mothers who breastfed initially (89%) received help or advice for these problems and almost all mothers talked to either a midwife or a nurse. Although it is a small group, mothers of first babies who said they did not get help in hospital were significantly more likely to have stopped breastfeeding by two weeks (50%) than those who had received help (28%).

Table 6.19

Problems feeding the baby after leaving hospital

Among mothers who were still breastfeeding when they left hospital, 35% reported having problems breastfeeding in the early weeks. Again, mothers of first babies were more likely to experience problems (40%) than mothers of second or later babies (30%).

Table 6.20

Table 6.19

Proportion of mothers who had stopped breastfeeding within two weeks by whether they received help with problems in hospital (United Kingdom 2000)

	First birth		Later births		All breastfed babies	
	Received help	Did not receive help	Received help	Did not receive help	Received help	Did not receive help
Percentage who had stopped breastfeeding within two weeks	28	50	31	41	29	47
Base (Stage 1 breastfeeding mothers having feeding problems in hospital)	1,276	126	547	80	1,820	205

Table 6.20

Feeding problems experienced by mothers after leaving hospital (1990, 1995 GB, 2000 UK)*

	First births			Later births			All breastfed babies		
	1990 %	1995 %	2000 %	1990 %	1995 %	2000 %	1990 %	1995 %	2000 %
Had problems	39	40	40	30	30	30	34	35	35
Did not have problems	61	60	60	70	70	69	66	65	64
Base (Stage 1 mothers breastfeeding when they left hospital)	1,377	1,407	2,761	1,480	1,464	2,797	2,857	2,878	5,558

* Note that 1990 and 1995 data based on GB, 2000 data based on UK

By this stage, the problems most frequently mentioned by breastfeeding mothers were that the mother had sore nipples (40%) and that the baby appeared hungry (32%). In addition, one quarter of breastfeeding mothers (24%) still reported problems with the baby rejecting the breast or not latching on. About one tenth (12%) of mothers who had feeding problems continued to say that the baby was prone to falling asleep or was slow feeding.

As found with problems experienced by mothers in hospital, bottle-feeding mothers were more likely than breastfeeding mothers to find that problems after hospital related to the health of their baby; this included vomiting (22% compared with 3% of breastfeeding mothers having problems after hospital) and colic (27% compared with 7%). Like breastfeeding mothers, a third (32%) of bottle-feeding mothers had problems with baby remaining unsatisfied after feeds and one in ten (10%) had problems with baby falling asleep/feeding too slowly or gaining insufficient weight.

Table 6.18

7.3 Reasons for stopping breastfeeding

Chapter 2 showed that one in six women (16%) in the UK who breastfed initially had given up within one week and one in five (21%) had given up within two weeks. After the initial two weeks (which have been considered in detail in Chapter 6), the rate of giving up breastfeeding slowed: two-thirds (64%) of mothers who had started breastfeeding were still doing so when their babies were six weeks old and one in three (34%) continued for six months or more. This section looks at the reasons cited by women for giving up breastfeeding and whether mothers would have liked to have breastfed for longer.

As shown in Table 7.10, the reasons for having given up varied with the duration of breastfeeding. In the early weeks reasons for giving up centred on problems with baby rejecting the breast (37% who gave up in the first week and 18% in the second), and painful nipples (27% and 28% of these mothers respectively). Mothers who tried breastfeeding for at least a week but gave up by the time their baby was 4 months were most likely to mention insufficient breastmilk as a reason for stopping. By 4 months, returning to work or college was beginning to become an important reason for stopping, especially so among mothers giving up between 4 and 6 months, with 39% stating this as a reason. From 6 months, the emergence of teeth was causing problems for some breastfeeding mothers (18%) and 19% of this subgroup of mothers said that it was simply the right time to stop.

Table 7.10

Table 7.10
Reasons given by mothers for stopping breastfeeding, by duration of breastfeeding (United Kingdom, 2000)

	Baby's age when breastfeeding ceased:					
	Less than 1 week %	1 week less than 2 weeks %	2 weeks less than 6 weeks %	6 weeks less than 4 months %	4 months less than 6 months %	6 months less than 9 months %
Baby rejected breast	37	18	13	10	12	15
Painful breasts/ nipples	27	28	23	8	2	1
Insufficient milk	26	40	53	52	30	21
Took too long/ tiring	12	16	24	17	8	4
Mother was ill	8	13	10	5	4	8
Didn't like breastfeeding	7	3	1	2	*	1
Baby was ill	6	12	6	4	2	2
Domestic reasons	3	9	11	6	2	1
Baby could not be fed by others	1	1	4	8	6	8
Returned to work/ college	1	-	2	19	39	27
Breastfed for as long as intended	*	*	1	4	6	5
Baby teething/ biting*				*	5	18
Time was right to stop*				-	8	19
Base *(Stage 3 mothers who stopped breastfeeding during survey period)*	*791*	*232*	*742*	*997*	*525*	*597*

Percentages do not add up to 100% as some mothers gave more than one answer
*code introduced at later waves of the survey

Whether mothers would have liked to breastfeed for longer

The reasons mothers gave for having stopped breastfeeding suggest that very few mothers gave up because they had planned to, particularly those stopping before four months. However, as a further measure, mothers who had given up breastfeeding were specifically asked whether they would have liked to have continued for longer. The vast majority of mothers who gave up within six weeks of birth – nine out of ten – would have liked to have breastfed for longer. Although this proportion declined with length of breastfeeding, it was still the case for two-thirds of mothers stopping between six weeks and four months, and for half of those stopping at four to six months. Even among those continuing to feed for at least six months, over a third would have liked to continue for longer. These results confirm the implications of the previous table, that women who start to breastfeed are generally committed to this method of feeding but are then deterred by problems or other circumstances.

Table 7.11

Table 7.11
Whether mothers would have liked to have breastfed longer,
by duration of breastfeeding (United Kingdom, 2000)

Baby's age when breastfeeding ceased	Would have liked to breastfeed longer	Base
	%	%
Less than 1 week	90	791
1 week, less than 2 weeks	93	232
2 weeks, less than 6 weeks	87	721
6 weeks, less than 4 months	69	997
4 months, less than 6 months	48	525
6 months or more	37	597

Base: Stage 3 breastfeeding mothers who stopped during the survey period

Whether mothers would breastfeed another baby

The mother's experience in breastfeeding her current baby was associated with her feeding intentions for future babies. Three in five mothers (62%) who had given up breastfeeding within the first week said that they would breastfeed another baby, with a quarter (27%) saying they would not. The comparable figures for mothers who had continued breastfeeding for at least six weeks were 97% who would breastfeed again, and just 1% who would not. So, mothers who had initially experienced difficulties with breastfeeding were, at this early stage, less inclined to repeat this experience if they had another child – although the majority would still do so.

Table 7.12

Table 7.12
Whether mothers would breastfeed another baby, by duration of breastfeeding
(United kingdom, 2000)

| If I had another baby: | Duration of breastfeeding | | | | |
	Less than 1 week %	1 week less than 2 weeks %	2 weeks less than 6 weeks %	6 weeks or more* %	All mothers** who breastfed %
- would breastfeed again	62	83	93	97	88
- would not breastfeed	27	14	4	1	7
- no answer given	11	3	3	2	4
Base	*791*	*232*	*742*	*3056*	*5020*
(Stage 3 mothers who breastfed initially)					

* Includes mothers still breastfeeding
** Includes some mothers where duration of breastfeeding not recorded

In Chapter 2, we saw that mothers who only fed their previous baby for a short period were more likely to breastfeed their subsequent baby in 2000, when compared to 1995. The results reported here suggest that mothers' future intentions, if they have another child, will follow the same trend. While overall there has been a small rise in the proportion of breastfeeding mothers who would repeat the experience, from 86% in 1995 to 88% in 2000, this increase is particularly marked amongst mothers who only breastfed for a short period, as Table 7.13 shows.

Table 7.13, Figure 7.2

Table 7.13
Whether mothers would breastfeed another baby, by duration of breastfeeding and survey year

| Would breastfeed again | Duration of breastfeeding | | | | |
	Less than 1 week %	1 week less than 2 weeks %	2 weeks less than 6 weeks %	6 weeks or more* %	All mothers** who breastfed %
1995 Survey	56	74	86	95	86
Base	*496*	*168*	*534*	*1961*	*3410*
(Stage 3 mothers who breastfed initially)					
2000 Survey	62	83	93	97	88
Base	*791*	*232*	*742*	*3056*	*5020*
(Stage 3 mothers who breastfed initially)					

* Includes mothers still breastfeeding
** Includes some mothers where duration of breastfeeding not recorded

Figure 7.2
Whether mothers would breastfeed another baby, by duration of breastfeeding within survey year

Base: All Stage 3 mothers who breastfed initially

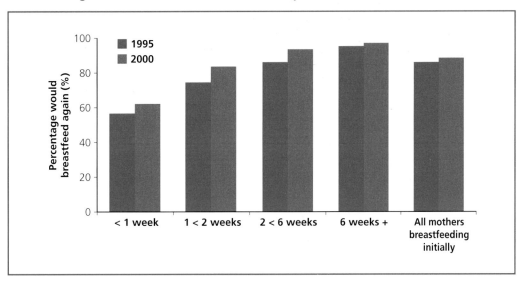

7.4 Employment status of mothers

As seen in the previous section, returning to work was one of the main reasons given by mothers who gave up breastfeeding from four months. Each stage of the Infant Feeding Survey included some questions about the mother's current employment status and the results are summarised here.

For the first stage of the survey, long-term trend data on mother's employment status is available. In 2000, when babies were about four to ten weeks old, almost half (46%) of all mothers were on paid maternity leave, a proportion which has been increasing steadily over the survey years (only 6% were on paid maternity leave at this stage in 1985). These shifts reflect changes in the sample composition of mothers over time as well as changes in maternity legislation, which has given more mothers access to paid maternity leave.

Table 7.14

Table 7.14

Mothers' working status when the babies were between 4 and 10 weeks old (1985, 1990, and 1995 Great Britain, and 2000 United Kingdom)

	Great Britain			United Kingdom
	1985 %	1990 %	1995 %	2000 %
Working	5	8	7	5
On maternity leave – paid	6	21	34	46
– unpaid	6	5	5	4
Not working	83	66	54	45
Base (All Stage 1 mothers)	*5223*	*5413*	*5017*	*9492*

For all stages, trend data are available for the last two survey years based on mothers in the United Kingdom. The significant rise between 1995 and 2000 in the proportion of mothers on maternity leave at stage 1 has already been noted. At Stage 2, there continues to be a significant rise between the survey years in the instance of mothers on maternity leave as opposed to non-working (22% in 2000 compared with 16% in 1995). By Stage 3, around half (49%) of mothers in 2000 were working, a small rise of 6 percentage points since 1995. The majority of the remainder were not working at all (48%), with only a negligible proportion (2%) still on maternity leave.

Table 7.15

Table 7.15

Mothers' working status at stages 1, 2 and 3, by survey year (United Kingdom)

	1995 %	2000 %
Stage 1 (4-10 weeks)		
Working	7	5
On maternity leave – paid	35	46
– unpaid	5	4
Not working	53	45
Base (All Stage 1 mothers)	*5181*	*9492*
Stage 2 (4-5 months)		
Working	28	27
On maternity leave – paid	4	9
– unpaid	12	13
Not working	56	50
Base (All Stage 2 mothers)	*5181*	*8299*
Stage 3 (8-9 months)		
Working	43	49
On maternity leave (paid or unpaid)	2	2
Not working	55	48
Base (All Stage 3 mothers)	*5181*	*7267*

In 2000, for the first time, mothers were asked in more detail about their working arrangements with a view to investigating whether there was a link between working patterns and how their baby was fed.

At Stage 3, the majority of working mothers were doing so part-time (up to 30 hours a week). About one in six (18%) were working less than 15 hours, with half (50%) working between 15 and 30 hours. Working mothers in Northern Ireland were more likely than working mothers in other countries to be doing so full-time (48% working 31 or more hours compared with 27% in England and Wales and 30% in Scotland). Mothers of first as opposed to later babies were also more likely to work full-time.

Table 7.16

Table 7.16
Number of hours worked per week by country and birth order (United Kingdom 2000)

	Country			Birth order		
	England & Wales %	Scotland %	Northern Ireland %	First baby %	Later baby %	All mothers %
No. hours worked/week						
Under 15	20	13	8	14	23	18
15-30	50	54	40	51	48	50
31+	27	30	48	31	25	28
Varies	2	2	2	2	3	2
Base (Stage 3 mothers at work)	*1976*	*943*	*762*	*1880*	*1667*	*3547*

Mothers were also asked about their childcare arrangements. Informal, unpaid childcare was the most commonly used form of childcare, with nearly half (46%) of mothers in the United Kingdom relying on the baby's grandparent(s) and a third (34%) using their partner. A childminder or nanny was used in one in five (19%) of cases where mothers were working and 15% used a non-workplace creche or nursery.

Compared with other countries, working mothers in Scotland made more use of the child's grandparents for childcare (54%) while working mothers in Northern Ireland were much less likely to use a husband or partner (19%), placing more reliance instead on childminders or nannies (26%).

Table 7.17

Table 7.17

Childcare used by mothers working at Stage 3 by country (United Kingdom, 2000)

	England & Wales	Scotland	Northern Ireland	United Kingdom
	%	%	%	%
Grandparent(s)	46	54	45	46
Husband or partner	35	33	19	34
Childminder/nanny	19	17	26	19
Creche or nursery (not workplace)	15	13	10	15
Another relative	8	11	12	9
Workplace creche or nursery	4	4	2	4
Friend	3	5	4	4
Other	1	*	-	1
Do not use childcare	4	4	3	4
Base (Mothers working at Stage 3)	*1976*	*943*	*762*	*3547*

Percentages do not add up to 100% as some mothers gave more than one answer

There was some variation in mothers' feeding behaviour by number of hours worked. Mothers working less than 15 hours were more likely than other working mothers to manage to provide milk solely from the breast (6% compared with 2% of those working full-time). Mothers working less than 15 hours were also twice as likely as mothers working full-time to manage to breastfeed at all (17% compared to 9%).

Table 7.18

Table 7.18

Milk feeding method at Stage 3 by mother's working hours (United Kingdom, 2000)

	Under 15 hours	15-30 hours	31+ hours	Hours vary	All working mothers*	All non-working mothers
	%	%	%	%	%	%
Breastmilk only	6	4	2	6	4	9
Breastmilk and other milk	11	7	7	3	7	6
No breastmilk given	83	89	90	92	89	85
Base (Mothers working at Stage 3)	*651*	*1763*	*1010*	*73*	*3547*	*3629*

Base includes some working mothers for whom hours not stated

There was very little difference between the feeding behaviours of mothers using different forms of childcare, although mothers using paid childcare (nursery/creche or childminder/nanny) were slightly more likely to give their baby mixed milk feeds (around one in ten of each group doing this) than mothers using other forms of childcare.

Table 7.19

Table 7.19
Milk feeding method at Stage 3 by mother's childcare arrangements (United Kingdom, 2000)

	Grand- parents	Husband/ partner	Child- minder/ nanny	Creche nursery	Other working mothers*	Do not use childcare
	%	%	%	%	%	%
Breastmilk only	3	5	2	3	3	6
Breastmilk and other milk	6	7	11	10	4	7
No breastmilk given	90	88	87	87	93	88
Base (Mothers working at Stage 3)	*1647*	*1192*	*673*	*643*	*441*	*128*

Mothers who were working at Stage 3 (when their babies were about eight or nine months old) were asked how their baby was provided with milk while they were at work. Just over half of this small subgroup (55%) gave their baby formula milk, while one in eight (12%) gave expressed breastmilk. The majority of the remainder (32%) opted to not give their baby any milk while they were at work. Mothers working part-time were less likely than full-time mothers to give formula milk (48% compared to 72%), instead being more likely to omit milk feeds altogether while at work (35% compared to 21%).

Table 7.20

Table 7.20
How baby was usually provided with milk while the mother was working, at stage 3 (United Kingdom, 2000)

	Working hours		All working mothers who breastfeed*
	Part-time (up to 30 hours) %	Full-time (31+ hours) %	%
Baby has formula milk	48	72	55
Baby has cows' milk	4	2	3
Baby has other milk (unspecified)	5	1	4
Baby not fed milk while mother at work	35	21	32
Baby has expressed breastmilk	12	13	12
Baby taken to work to breastfeed	3	2	4
Mother breastfeeds baby at lunchtime	2	2	2
Other arrangement	3	1	3
Base (Working mothers breastfeeding at stage 3)	*248*	*88*	*343*

Percentages do not add up to 100% as some mothers gave more than one answer
* Base includes some mothers for whom working hours either varied or were not stated

Mothers who were working at Stage 3 were asked specifically whether their return to work had affected the way they fed their baby. Overall one in six (16%) said that this was the case. Working mothers in Scotland were slightly more likely than mothers in other countries to have found this (19% compared with 16% in England and Wales and 13% in Northern Ireland).

There was also a greater propensity for feeding practices to be affected by work among mothers working full as opposed to part-time, and among mother in higher occupations, as shown in Table 7.21.

Table 7.21

Table 7.21
Whether return to work has affected the way mothers feed their babies by working hours and mother's socio-economic group (NS-SEC) (United Kingdom 2000)

Base: Mothers working at Stage 3	Proportion saying baby's feeding affected	Base
	%	%
Part-time (up to 30 hours)	13	2415
Full-time (31+ hours)	24	1010
Higher occupations	25	1577
Intermediate occupations	10	871
Lower occupations*	7	791
Never worked	9	108
Unclassified	13	200
All working mothers*	16	3547

** Base includes some mothers for whom working hours varied or were not stated

Mothers who said their baby's feeding had been affected by work were asked in what ways. Answers were collected as an open response and later coded. The responses given by mothers are provided in Table 7.22. In the large majority of cases (71%), the reason was linked to cutting down or cessation of breastfeeding, and this confirms the findings reported in section 7.3 which also showed how working was a major reason for mothers having to give up this method of feeding. Other changes mentioned by smaller proportions were having less time to prepare home-made solid food (10%) and changing baby's feeding routine (10%).

Table 7.22

Table 7.22
How return to work has affected feeding of baby (United Kingdom 2000)

	%
Stopped or cut down breastfeeding	71
Less time to prepare home-made foods	10
Change to baby's feeding routine	10
Less control over baby's diet	4
Ensure baby weaned onto solids before returned to work	2
Other	3
Base (All mothers working at stage 3 who say that baby's feeding been affected)	573

7.5 Contact with health professionals

As part of the stage one questionnaire, mothers were asked whether a health visitor had been to see them since their baby was born and, if so, how old the baby was at the first visit. Nearly all mothers (99%) had seen a health visitor by the time they completed the questionnaire when their baby was four to ten weeks old. Their babies were, on average, 12 days old at the time of the first visit, with three-quarters of all first visits occurring when the baby was between six and fifteen days old. Results on this measure were similar across the three countries.

Table 7.23

Table 7.23
Age of baby when health visitor first visited mother and baby, by country (2000)

	England & Wales	Scotland	Northern Ireland	United Kingdom
	%	%	%	%
Up to 5 days old	6	7	9	6
6-10 days	35	36	35	35
11-15 days	41	45	40	41
16-20 days	8	5	7	8
21+ days	7	4	5	7
Mean age of baby (days)	**12.2**	**11.3**	**11.6**	**12.1**
Base *(Babies who had been visited* *by Stage 1)*	*5368*	*2247*	*1761*	*9376*

Nearly half (47%) of mothers said that their baby had had a development check-up by stage one of the survey. However, it should be noted that the age of babies at Stage 1 varied from 3 to 18 weeks (see Table 2.25), and whether mothers had received developmental check-ups varied considerably by their baby's age at the time of completing the stage 1 survey. For example, only a fifth (20%) of mothers with babies aged less than 6 weeks at Stage 1 had received such a check-up, rising to a half (47%) of mothers with babies aged 6 up to 8 weeks, and nearly all (82%) of mothers with babies aged 8 weeks or more at Stage 1.

In the United Kingdom, around half of all check-ups (56%) took place at the general practitioner's, with a further quarter (24%) taking place at a child health clinic or hospital. The remaining one-fifth (19%) took place at the family home. Compared with other mothers, mothers in Northern Ireland were more likely to have home-based checks, and less likely to have checks based at the doctor's surgery. Compared with 1995, more mothers are now having home visits (in the UK 19% compared to 8% in 1995).

Table 7.24

Table 7.24
Location of developmental check-up by country (2000)

	England & Wales		Scotland		Northern Ireland		United Kingdom	
	1995 %	2000 %	1995 %	2000 %	1995 %	2000 %	1995 %	2000 %
Child health clinic/ hospital	30	23	35	30	31	24	31	24
Family doctor/ GP	62	57	61	60	41	42	61	56
At home	8	19	4	10	27	34	8	19
Base (Stage 1 mothers who had had developmental check-up)	*2910*	*2431*	*1644*	*1345*	*1024*	*1265*	*3393*	*4473*

At stage two of the survey, when babies were four or five months old, mothers were asked if they took their baby to a child health clinic or to their general practitioner for advice or regular check-ups. Almost nine out of ten (87%) said they took their baby to the child health clinic, and a third (33%) took their baby to their general practitioner, with 91% saying they took their baby to at least one of the two for advice or check-ups.

Mothers in Northern Ireland were less likely to go to a child health clinic (74%) and more likely to go to their general practitioner (43%) than mothers in England and Wales or Scotland. Results are similar for the two survey years.

Table 7.25

Table 7.25
Whether mother took baby to child health clinic or general practitioner for advice or regular check-ups, by country and survey year (stage 2)

	England & Wales		Scotland		Northern Ireland		United Kingdom	
	1995 %	2000 %	1995 %	2000 %	1995 %	2000 %	1995 %	2000 %
Took baby to child health clinic	87	88	87	88	71	74	86	87
Took baby to family doctor/GP	36	33	35	29	45	43	36	33
Base (Stage 2 mothers)	*4589*	*4729*	*1861*	*1953*	*1473*	*1618*	*5181*	*8299*

Most mothers in the United Kingdom took their baby to the child health clinic either about once a fortnight (34%) or about once a month (45%). As well as being less likely to visit a child health clinic, mothers in Northern Ireland also tended to visit less frequently. A fifth (22%) visited with a frequency of at least fortnightly compared with nearly half (45%) in England and Wales.

Visits to the general practitioner for those who made them were a much less routine affair, with half (51%) making visits less than once a month, although mothers in Northern

Ireland making visits did so with a greater frequency (46% visiting monthly compared with 31% and 37% of the equivalent subgroups in Scotland and England and Wales).

Table 7.26

Table 7.26
How often mother took baby to child health clinic or general practitioner for advice or regular check-ups at Stage 2 by country (2000)

	England & Wales	Scotland	Northern Ireland	United Kingdom
	%	%	%	%
Frequency of attending child health clinic				
Once a week	10	6	5	9
Once a fortnight	35	28	17	34
Once a month	44	48	54	45
Less than once a month	11	17	23	12
Base:	*4146*	*1713*	*1193*	*7214*
(Stage 2 mothers who attended child health clinic)				
Frequency of visiting GP				
Once a week	2	1	1	2
Once a fortnight	7	7	5	7
Once a month	37	31	46	38
Less than once a month	51	57	45	51
Base:				
(Stage 2 mothers who visited GP)	*1541*	*576*	*694*	*2734*

There was no change from 1995 in the frequency of attendance at child health clinics or at the general practitioners. However, within the 2000 data, there was a difference in the frequency of attendance at child health clinics by birth order. Although nearly all mothers of both first (91%) and later births (84%) took their child to these clinics, mothers of first babies who made such visits did so with a much greater frequency. Over half (53%) of first-time mothers took their babies at least fortnightly compared with a third (34%) of mothers with later babies.

Mothers of first and later babies were equally likely to make GP visits (32% and 33% respectively) and there was relatively little difference in the frequency of visits made by these mothers.

Table 7.27

145

Table 7.29
Where mothers prefer to feed when in a public place by mother's socio-economic group (NS-SEC (United Kingdom 2000)

	Higher occupations	Intermediate occupations	Lower occupations	Never worked	Unclassified working	All mothers
	%	%	%	%	%	%
Have breastfed in public	**92**	**91**	**89**	**73**	**90**	**90**
Prefer mother & baby room	45	45	45	41	47	45
Prefer to breastfeed without going to special place	22	20	14	9	16	19
No preference	25	25	30	22	26	26
Never breastfed in public place	**8**	**9**	**11**	**27**	**9**	**10**
Base (Mothers breastfeeding at Stage 2)	*1026*	*461*	*362*	*167*	*177*	*2193*

Finally, all mothers at stage 2 were asked where they thought it was important to have facilities for feeding babies, and three places were specifically prompted in the question - shops/ shopping centres, restaurants, and public toilets. Nearly all mothers (94%) said they thought shops and shopping centres should provide facilities, four-fifths (79%) mentioned restaurants, and a third (34%) thought there should be feeding facilities in public toilets. A small number of mothers also spontaneously suggested travel terminals and places of entertainment such as parks and museums. There were no substantial differences by either feeding method or survey year.

Table 7.30

Table 7.30
Places that mothers thought should provide facilities for feeding babies, by feeding method and survey year (Great Britain 1995, United Kingdom 2000)*

	Breastfeeders		Bottle feeders		All mothers	
	1995 %	2000 %	1995 %	2000 %	1995 %	2000 %
Shops/ shopping centres	98	95	96	93	97	94
Restaurants	78	77	81	80	80	79
Public toilets	41	37	31	33	33	34
Stations and airports	6	2	2	*	3	1
Places of leisure/entertainment	7	4	4	1	5	2
Other public places	7	7	4	3	4	4
Base (Stage 2 mothers)	*1224*	*2195*	*3733*	*6073*	*4957*	*8299*

Percentages do not add up to 100% as some mothers gave more than one answer
* Note that 1995 data is based on Great Britain

8

Additional drinks and supplementary vitamins

Summary

- Just over half (55%) of mothers were giving their baby drinks other than milk at four to ten weeks. Mothers who were bottle feeding were more likely to have introduced other drinks (76%) than women who were breastfeeding (27%).

- Water was the most commonly mentioned additional drink at all three stages. Compared with 1995 results, there has been a marked shift away from sweetened drinks to unsweetened drinks, and from all other types of drinks to unsweetened water.

- Mothers from higher socio-economic groups were less likely than mothers in lower groups or who had never worked to be giving additional drinks at both the four to ten weeks and four to five months stages of the survey.

- The majority of mothers (85%) had introduced their baby to a cup by the final stage of survey when their babies were aged eight to nine months. Compared with 1995, mothers were introducing a cup earlier in 2000.

- At four to ten weeks, just 4% of babies received additional vitamins, 5% at four to five months and 10% at eight to nine months. These figures continue a longer-term trend in the declining use of this practice over the survey years. Babies of low birthweight, and babies born to mothers of Black or Asian parents were more likely than average to be receiving vitamins.

- A third (35%) of breastfeeding mothers were taking supplementary vitamins and/ or iron tablets at stage one, falling to just over a quarter at the four and nine month stages (27% and 26% respectively). At all three stages of the survey, breastfeeding mothers in Northern Ireland were more likely than mothers in other countries to have taken supplementary vitamins.

This chapter covers the provision of drinks to babies at all three stages of the survey, how many mothers are giving drinks and the types of drinks given. We also investigate the practice of giving supplementary vitamins to babies, as well as the level of women who take supplementary vitamins themselves.

8.1 Additional drinks

The Department of Health recommends that there is no need to give drinks other than breast milk or infant formula for the first four to six months of life. The Committee On Medical Aspects of Food Policy (COMA) Report on Weaning and the Weaning Diet[1] recommends that cooled boiled water to satisfy thirst between feeds or diluted fruit juices at meal times are suitable when the older baby is being weaned onto solid foods.

8.1.1 Proportion of mothers giving additional drinks

At each stage of the survey, mothers were asked whether they were giving their baby any drinks additional to milk – including water or other drinks. In the United Kingdom, just over half (55%) of mothers were giving their baby drinks other than milk at the first stage of the survey, when babies were about 4-10 weeks old.

Mothers who were bottle-feeding their babies at Stage 1 were much more likely than mothers who were breastfeeding at this stage to have introduced additional drinks (76% compared with 27%). Compared with 1995, results have remained broadly similar, although the differential between breast and bottle-feeding mothers has widened somewhat since 1995.

Table 8.1

Table 8.1
Additional drinks given to babies at stage 1, by method of feeding (Great Britain 1995*, United Kingdom 2000)

	Breastfeeding at Stage 1		Bottle-feeding at Stage 1		All Stage 1 mothers	
	GB 1995* %	UK 2000 %	GB 1995* %	UK 2000 %	UK 1995 %	UK 2000 %
Drinks given	30	27	69	76	54	55
Base	1954	4004	3063	5459	5181	9492

* 1995 data on bottle and breastfeeding mothers only available at GB level

Table 8.2 shows the proportion of mothers giving additional drinks at Stages 1 and 2 of the survey by country. At Stage 1 the proportion of babies receiving drinks other than milk was notably higher in Northern Ireland (70%) compared with other countries. Additionally this figure has risen slightly from 1995 (64%), while rates in other countries have remained stable.

By Stage 2, the large majority of mothers were giving additional drinks - around three-quarters (74%) in the United Kingdom, slightly higher in Northern Ireland (78%). Overall at the United Kingdom level, there has been a slight reduction in the proportion giving extra drinks at Stage 2 (from 77% to 74%).

Table 8.2

Table 8.2
Proportions of mothers giving drinks other than milk at stages 1 and 2, by country (1995 and 2000 United Kingdom)

	England & Wales		Scotland		Northern Ireland		United Kingdom	
	1995	2000	1995	2000	1995	2000	1995	2000
At 4-10 weeks	54	54	55	54	64	70	54	55
Base: All stage 1 mothers	4598	5440	1863	2274	1476	1778	5181	9492
At four to five months	76	73	77	75	80	78	77	74
Base: All stage 2 mothers	4598	4729	1863	1953	1476	1617	5181	8299

The proportion of mothers giving drinks to their babies varied by mother's socio-economic group. Mothers classified into higher socio-economic groups were less likely than mothers in lower groups or who had never worked to give drinks in addition to milk. At Stage 1, two-fifths (40%) of mothers classified to higher occupations were giving drinks compared with around two-thirds of mothers in lower occupations or who had never worked. A similar differential occurred at Stage 2 with two-thirds (64%) of mothers in higher occupations giving drinks compared with eight in ten mothers in lower occupations or who had never worked.

Table 8.3, Figure 8.1

Table 8.3
Proportions of mothers giving drinks other than milk at stages 1 and 2 by mother's socio-economic classification (NS-SEC) (United Kingdom, 2000)

	Higher occupations	Intermediate occupations	Lower occupations	Never worked	Unclassi-fied
At 4-10 weeks	40	52	66	69	57
Base: All stage 1 mothers	2790	1905	2619	1276	901
At four to five months	64	72	81	82	79
Base: All stage 2 mothers	2546	1740	2286	979	749

Figure 8.1

Proportions of mothers giving drinks other than milk at stages 1 and 2 by mother's socio-economic classification (NS-SEC) (United Kingdom, 2000)

Base: All mothers

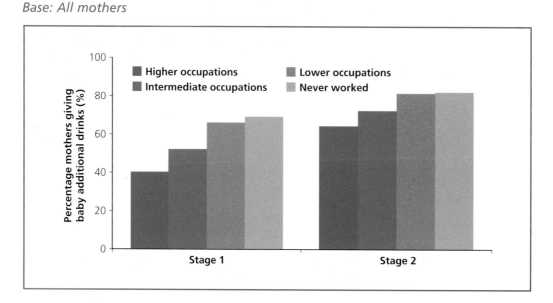

8.1.2 Types of drinks given

Table 8.4 shows the types of drinks given to babies at each of the stages of the survey, in addition to milk. It should be noted that the categories 'baby drink, unsweetened' and 'adult drink, unsweetened' means no *added* sugar. Thus, these categories could include drinks in which sugars are present naturally, for example fruit juice. Appendix V gives examples of the types of drinks included in each of the categories.

At all three stages, plain water was by far the most common type of drink (other than milk) which mothers were giving. Half (54%) of all stage 1 mothers had given water, rising to two thirds (65%) at stage 2 and four fifths (83%) at stage 3. Indeed, at stage 1 very few mothers gave any additional drinks other than water. In particular, less than half a percent mentioned any of the categories of sweetened drinks (2% gave unsweetened baby drinks, and 2% gave commercial herbal drinks).

By the time the babies were around four to five months, the proportion of mothers giving unsweetened baby drinks had risen to one third (33%) – water was still twice as commonly given. Sweetened drinks of all types were still relatively uncommon, although when specifically prompted, 5% said that they sometimes gave their baby water that had been sweetened with honey or sugar.

At eight to nine months, the proportion providing their baby with unsweetened baby drinks remained at around a third (35%), although adult drinks were starting to become more common. Although in half of these cases insufficient information was given to say whether the adult drink was sweetened or not, in the large majority of cases where this information was given, the drink was unsweetened. One in six (16%) of all mothers gave unsweetened adult drinks; one in five (20%) gave adult drinks that could not be specified from the information supplied.

At all three stages, compared with 1995 results, there has been a definite shift away from sweetened to unsweetened drinks, and significantly more mothers are giving just plain water. In particular, in 1995 unsweetened baby drinks were more commonly given than water at stages 2 and 3, a situation which has reversed in 2000. At Stage 3 a quarter of mothers in 1995 were giving their baby adult drinks with sugar or glucose and one in six adult drinks with artificial sweetener, these figures reducing to negligible levels in 2000. There has also been a move away from herbal drinks compared with 1995 (this practice was quite prevalent in 1990 but has dropped away to almost negligible levels over the ten years since).

Table 8.4

Table 8.4

Types of drink given at stages 1, 2 and 3 of the survey (1995 Great Britain, 2000 United Kingdom)

	Stage 1 (4-10 weeks)		Stage 2 (4-5 months)		Stage 3 (8-9 months)	
	1995*	2000	1995*	2000	1995*	2000
Plain or mineral water	39	54	41	65	59	83
Water with sugar/ honey added**	7	*	4	5	3	2
Baby drink with sugar/ glucose	1	*	3	1	3	1
Baby drink unsweetened=	9	2	63	33	76	35
Herbal drink	8	2	9	2	5	1
Adult drink with sugar/ glucose	1	*	3	*	23	3
Adult drink with artificial sweetener	-	*	1	*	16	1
Adult drink unsweetened†	2	1	8	4	21	16
Adult drink unspecified	-	*	1	2	-	20
Other drink	2	2	2	2	2	3
Base (All mothers at relevant stage)	*5017*	*9492*	*5017*	*8299*	*5017*	*7267*

Percentages do not add up to 100% as some mothers gave more than one answer
See Appendix V for coding frame
* Note that 1995 results are based on GB data and 2000 results based on UK data
**Specific question about addition of sugar and honey not asked at stage 1
† no added sweetener

Looking at the simpler breakdown of mothers giving water and drinks other than water, a clear pattern according to mother's socio-economic group emerges. At both stages 1 and 2, mothers at the higher end of the socio-economic classification were less likely to give both water and other drinks compared to mothers at the lower end. For example, at Stage 1, 40% of mothers in higher occupations were giving water compared with 68% of mothers who had never worked. Mothers who had never worked were also three times more likely to be giving "other" drinks than mothers in higher occupations (12% compared to 4%). Similar differentials are evident at Stage 2.

Table 8.5

Table 8.5

Proportions of mothers giving water and other drinks additional to milk at stages 1 and 2 by mother's socio-economic classification (NS-SEC) (United Kingdom, 2000)

	Higher occupations	Intermediate occupations	Lower occupations	Never worked	Unclassi-fied
At 4-10 weeks					
Giving water	40	51	65	68	56
Giving other drinks	4	7	11	12	8
Base: All stage 1 mothers	*2790*	*1905*	*2619*	*1276*	*901*
At four to five months					
Giving water	57	65	71	70	69
Giving other drinks	30	36	51	55	44
Base: All stage 2 mothers	*2546*	*1740*	*2286*	*979*	*749*

8.1.3 Reasons for giving additional drinks

The most common reason stated for giving the baby additional drinks at both four to ten weeks and at four to five months was that the mother thought the baby was thirsty between feeds. Three in five (62%) of mothers giving additional drinks at stage 1, and four in five (82%) at stage 2 gave this reason.

At Stage 1, drinks were also given quite commonly to aid against constipation (55%), colic (33%) or just to settle the baby (28%). By Stage 2, constipation and colic were less of an issue for mothers giving drinks (27% and 8% respectively).

The reasons mothers cite for giving their babies additional drinks also varies by the method of feeding. At both stages, bottle-feeding mothers who gave additional drinks were more likely than breastfeeding mothers to do so because they thought their baby to be thirsty between feeds. Bottle-feeding mothers giving drinks were also slightly more likely to say that this was to settle their baby (although this difference was only significant at Stage 2). On the other hand, at Stage 1, breastfeeding mothers were more likely than bottle-feeders to say they gave extra drinks to help with baby's colic or digestion.

Table 8.6

8.1.4 Use of a cup or beaker

The Weaning and the Weaning Diet Report[1] recommends that 'from six months of age, infants should be introduced to drinking from a cup' to reduce long term bottle-use and improve dental health. When they were aged about nine months old, six out of seven (85%) babies had drunk from a cup or beaker with a spout. Babies in Scotland were more likely to have done so (89%) than those in Northern Ireland (85%) or England and Wales (84%). Compared with 1995, there was a slight rise in the level reporting use of a cup (from 78% to 85%) and a similar rise could be found in all countries.

Table 8.7

Table 8.6

Reasons for giving additional drinks at stages 1 and 2 of the survey by method of feeding at that stage (United Kingdom 2000)

	4-10 weeks (Stage 1)			4-5 months (Stage 2)		
	Breast %	Bottle %	All babies* %	Breast %	Bottle %	All babies* %
Because baby is thirsty	39	66	62	65	85	82
To help baby's constipation	48	57	55	26	27	27
To help baby's colic/ wind/ digestion	46	32	33	7	8	8
To settle the baby	22	29	28	15	21	20
To give baby extra vitamins	6	7	7	11	13	13
Other reason	2	4	4	23	8	10
Base (Mothers giving babies additional drinks other than water)	*103*	*625*	*738*	*497*	*2917*	*3431*

Percentages do not add up to 100% as some mothers gave more than one answer
* Includes some babies for whom method of feeding not known

Table 8.7

Whether baby had ever drunk from a cup or beaker by 8 to 9 months (United Kingdom, 1995 & 2000)

	England & Wales		Scotland		Northern Ireland		United Kingdom	
	1995 %	2000 %	1995 %	2000 %	1995 %	2000 %	1995 %	2000 %
	78	84	86	89	81	85	78	85
Base: All stage 3 mothers	*4598*	*4111*	*1863*	*1719*	*1497*	*1437*	*5181*	*7267*

Table 8.8 and Figure 8.2 show the age at which babies who had used a cup or beaker first did so. In 2000, half (49%) of babies in the United Kingdom using a cup had used one by the age of six months. Seven in ten (70%) of all babies using a cup had done so by the age of seven months.

Mothers introducing a cup were doing so earlier in 2000 than in 1995. A quarter (26%) had introduced the cup by 5 months compared with one in seven (15%) in 1995. By seven months, the differential is 70% (2000) against 61% (1995).

Table 8.8, Figure 8.2

Table 8.8
Age by which babies had used a cup or beaker with a spout (1995 & 2000, United Kingdom)

	1995	2000
	%	%
4 months	7	11
5 months	15	26
6 months	36	49
7 months	61	70
8 months*	77	84
9 months*	96	93
10 months+*	100	100
Base (Stage 3 babies who had ever used a cup)	*3927*	*6154*

*In 2000, based on reduced number of cases excluding those babies who had not reached this age by Stage 3

Figure 8.2
Age by which babies had used a cup or beaker with a spout (1995 & 2000, United Kingdom)

Base: All Stage 3 babies ever used cup

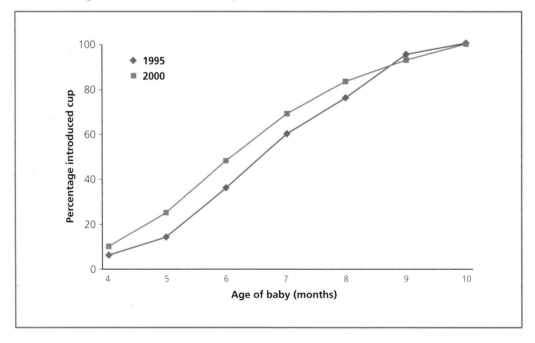

Babies of mothers classified to higher socio-economic groups were more likely to have used a cup or beaker by the age of six months compared to mothers in lower socio-economic groups. Nearly half (45%) of mothers in the higher occupational group had introduced their baby to a cup by 6 months, compared to a third (32%) of mothers who had never worked.

Table 8.9

Table 8.9
Proportion of mothers who had introduced their baby to a cup by 6 months by mother's socio-economic group (NS-SEC) (United Kingdom, 2000)

	Higher occupations	Intermediate occupations	Lower occupations	Never worked	Unclassi-fied
Introduced cup by 6 months	45	42	38	32	40
Base: All stage 3 mothers	*2315*	*1558*	*1982*	*769*	*643*

8.2 Supplementary vitamins

Certain infants such as premature babies or babies of mothers with vitamin deficiencies may not be receiving required levels of nutrients through breast or formula milks. They may require the early use of supplements of Vitamins A, C and D. Otherwise, the COMA Report on Weaning and the Weaning Diet[1] recommends that vitamin supplements should be given to children aged from six months. Babies who are consuming 500ml of infant formula or follow-on formula a day do not need vitamin supplementation because these products are fortified. (The use of vitamin C enriched fruit drinks to aid iron absorption is discussed separately in Chapter 9.)

8.2.1 Use of vitamins for the baby

The proportion of babies in 2000 being given vitamins at four to ten weeks is just 4%. This continues a longer-term trend in declining use of this practice. In 1985, nearly three in ten babies in Great Britain (27%) were receiving extra vitamins at the time of the Stage 1 survey, which fell to 6% by 1995. By Stage 2, the level of mothers in 2000 giving extra vitamins remained similar to the level at Stage 1 (5%), this also continuing a longer-term decline. Table 8.7 shows the data from 1990 onwards.

Table 8.10

Table 8.10
Whether supplementary vitamins given to babies at Stage 1 and Stage 2 (United Kingdom, 1990, 1995, & 2000)

	1990	1995	2000
	%	%	%
At four to ten weeks	12	6	4
Base: All Stage 1 mothers	*5533*	*5181*	*9492*
At four to five months	19	10	5
Base: All Stage 2 mothers	*5533*	*5181*	*8298*

The data for Stages 1 and 2 showed no difference by feeding method. However, there were some groups of mothers who were more likely than average to be giving vitamins at Stage 1. These included mothers of babies who began life in special care (26% giving vitamins), babies of low birthweight under 2500g (36% giving vitamins), and babies of Asian or Black parentage (11% and 17% respectively). The latter two findings are related since babies born to Black or Asian mothers are smaller on average compared with white babies. Also, babies born to Asian mothers are advised to give drops containing Vitamin D. The higher prevalence of giving vitamins among these groups continues at Stage 2.

Table 8.11

Table 8.11
Whether supplementary vitamins given to babies at Stage 1 and Stage 2 by special care, birth weight and ethnicity (United Kingdom, 2000)

	Baby in special care		Baby's birthweight				Ethnicity			
	Yes %	No %	< 2500g %	2500-3499g %	3500g + %	White %	Black %	Asian %	Mixed %	Other
At 4 to 10 weeks	26	2	36	2	2	3	11	17	5	–
Base: All Stage 1 mothers	846	8551	539	4766	4093	8608	275	184	93	67
At 4 to 5 months	24	3	35	3	3	4	23	17	8	4
Base: All Stage 2 mothers	713	7507	447	4162	3640	7631	202	132	80	57

By Stage 3, there was an increase in the proportion of mothers from the 2000 survey giving extra vitamins, with one in ten (10%) doing so. This again represents a declining trend over the survey years (30% in 1990 and 17% in 1995 - these figures based on mothers in Great Britain).

At Stage 3, there was a variation in the level of mothers giving vitamins by method of milk feeding. Breastfeeding mothers and those giving liquid cow's milk were the most likely to be giving vitamins (18% and 17% respectively), while those giving formula feeds were the least likely (8%).

Table 8.12

Table 8.12
Whether supplementary vitamins given to babies at about 8 to 9 months old, by feeding method (United Kingdom 2000)

	Breastfed	Bottle fed		All babies*
	%	Liquid cow's milk %	Infant formula %	%
Received vitamins	18	17	8	10
Base (All Stage 3 mothers)	959	538	5752	7266
*includes some babies who received only non-human milk for which type was not known				

There was relatively little difference in the proportion of mothers giving vitamins by country, although babies in Northern Ireland were slightly less likely than babies in other countries to be receiving vitamins at stages 2 and 3. The decrease in proportions over time within country reflect the general trend in declining use of vitamins as discussed above.

Table 8.13

Table 8.13

Proportion of mothers giving extra vitamins at stages 1, 2 and 3, by country (1995 and 2000 United Kingdom)

	England & Wales		Scotland		Northern Ireland		United Kingdom	
	1995 %	2000 %	1995 %	2000 %	1995 %	2000 %	1995 %	2000 %
At four to ten weeks	6	4	8	3	3	3	6	4
At four to five months	9	5	13	6	8	3	10	5
At eight to nine months	n/a*	11	n/a*	9	n/a*	7	n/a*	10
Bases:								
Stage 1 mothers	*4598*	*5440*	*1863*	*2275*	*1476*	*1778*	*5181*	*9492*
Stage 2 babies	*4598*	*4729*	*1863*	*1953*	*1476*	*1618*	*5181*	*8299*
Stage 3 babies		*4112*		*1719*		*1438*		*7266*

* Data not available for 1995

Of those who were giving vitamin drops at any of the three stages, two thirds at each stage used Department of Health Children's Vitamin Drops that they either bought, or received free or on prescription from the Child Health Clinic. At four to ten weeks, mothers were more likely to receive their vitamins free of charge or on prescription; at later stages the mothers were more likely to buy their babies' vitamins. Over three in five mothers giving vitamins at stage one received them free or on prescription, falling to two in five at stage two and one in five at stage three.

Table 8.14

Table 8.14

Types of vitamins given at stages 1, 2 and 3 (United Kingdom 2000)

	4-10 weeks	4-5 months	8-9 months
	%	%	%
Children's Vitamin Drops:	64	66	68
Bought at a clinic	13	22	34
Free/ prescribed at clinic	43	28	17
Obtained elsewhere	7	14	18
Other brands:	31	35	31
Bought	9	18	29
Prescribed	22	15	2
Base (Mothers giving supplementary vitamins)	*363*	*425*	*743*

8.2.2 Use of vitamins for the mother

"Present day practice in infant feeding: third report"[2] states that the vitamin content of human milk is sufficient for the infant's requirements provided the mother has a balanced diet. At about four to ten weeks, a third (35%) of breastfeeding mothers were taking supplementary vitamins and/ or iron tablets, this falling to around a quarter over the next two survey stages.

By country, it emerges that breastfeeding mothers in Northern Ireland were more likely than these mothers in other countries to have taken supplementary vitamins. Around two-fifths (43%) were taking vitamins at Stage 1 compared with around a third (34%) in England and Wales and Scotland. This differential remained at Stages 2 and 3 with a third of breastfeeding mothers in Northern Ireland taking vitamins at Stage 3 compared to about a quarter in the other countries.

Table 8.15, Figure 8.3

Table 8.15

Percentage of breastfeeding mothers who took supplementary vitamins at stages 1, 2 and 3, by country, 2000

	England & Wales	Scotland	Northern Ireland	United Kingdom
	%	%	%	%
At four to ten weeks	34	34	43	35
At four to five months	27	24	34	27
At eight to nine months	26	23	34	26
Bases				
All breastfeeding mothers at Stage 1	*2374*	*897*	*421*	*3692*
All breastfeeding mothers at Stage 2	*1289*	*518*	*212*	*2019*
All breastfeeding mothers at Stage 3	*561*	*232*	*80*	*873*

Figure 8.3

Percentage of breastfeeding mothers who took supplementary vitamins at stages 1, 2 and 3, by country, 2000

Base: All breastfeeding mothers

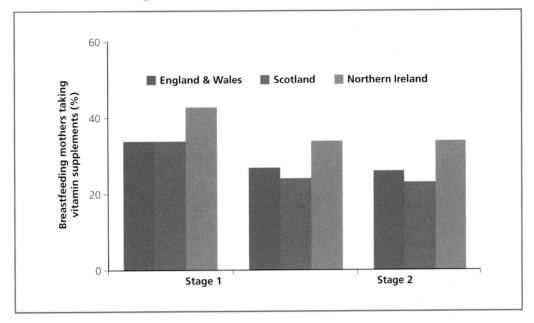

[1] Department of Health. *Weaning and the Weaning Diet, Report of the Working Group on the Weaning Diet of the Committee on Medical Aspects of Food Policy* Report on Health and Social Subjects 45, HMSO (London:1994)

[2] Department of Health and Social Security. *Present day practice in infant feeding: third report.* Report on Health and Social Subjects 32. HMSO (London: 1988)

9

Solid foods

Age of introduction of solid foods

- Compared with 1995, mothers in 2000 were introducing solids later. By three months, a quarter of mothers (24%) had introduced solid foods, which was less than half the proportion recorded in 1995 (56%). The majority (85%) had introduced solids by the age of four months and by six months, virtually all babies had been introduced to solid food.

- Despite this movement towards later introduction of solids, a high proportion of mothers was starting solid food earlier than thought desirable. Only half (49%) of mothers had introduced solids within the recommended window of four to six months (16 to 26 weeks), the large majority of the remainder introducing solids before 16 weeks (49% of all mothers).

- Solid food tended to be introduced at a younger age amongst mothers in Northern Ireland, mothers of babies with heavier birth weights, those in lower social classes, and mothers with lower educational levels. In addition, white mothers introduced solids earlier on average than mothers of Asian, Black and mixed ethnic origins.

Solid foods given at different ages

- When babies were four to five months old, mothers giving solids were more likely to give commercially prepared babyfood (62%) than home-made food (38%), although by eight to nine months this had reversed, with seven in ten mothers (70%) giving home-made food compared with 52% giving babyfood.

- Six per cent of mothers said they had never given their baby meat: of these, three in five said it was because their baby was not ready for it yet, and three in ten said they intended to give their baby a vegetarian diet. Concern about BSE appears to have abated since 1995, with results for meat consumption returning to the levels of the 1990 survey.

Influences on choice of solid food

- In choosing which solid foods to give their baby, mothers at stage two most frequently took account of the nutritional value of foods, either in general terms or specifically relating to sugar, vitamins, gluten or salt. The desire to give baby a variety of flavours and food that suited their preferences were also taken into account

- Half (47%) of stage three mothers avoided particular ingredients, most commonly sugar, salt and nuts. The most common reason for avoiding ingredients was allergies – this being a reason for a third (35%) of avoidances.

Difficulties with weaning

- One in ten mothers said that they had encountered difficulties in weaning their child onto solid foods, a half attributing this to their baby only accepting certain types of food. Compared with white mothers, mothers from ethnic minority backgrounds were much more likely to report problems with feeding their baby solids.

In this chapter, we explore the age of introduction of solid food, how this varies by different subgroups, and trends over time. We also investigate the different types of food given by mothers to their babies at different ages, influences on mothers' choice of solid food and any difficulties encountered.

9.1   Age of introduction of solid food

The COMA Report of the Working Group on the Weaning Diet1 recommends that 'the majority of infants should not be given solid foods before the age of four months, and a mixed diet should be offered by six months'. In 2001, the WHO issued a revised global recommendation that mothers should breastfeed exclusively for 6 months. Mothers in the 2000 survey will clearly not have been exposed to this advice as the survey predates it. However, it is useful to look at the 2000 figures in the light of these recommendations so that a benchmark can be set for tracking trends in later surveys.

9.1.1   Trend data by country

The results over time have shown that, in each subsequent survey wave, the age of introduction of solids has become progressively later[2]. This has tended to reflect changes in the recommendations prevailing at the time of the different surveys, as well as changes in the composition of the samples of mothers. In 2000, a very small proportion of mothers in the UK (3%) had introduced solid foods by the time their babies were six weeks old, which was lower than the proportion recorded in 1995 (7%). By three months, a quarter (24%) had already introduced solids, less than half the proportion recorded in 1995 (56%). These figures indicate a declining trend in early weaning although a significant proportion are still introducing solid foods early.

By country, it can be seen that mothers in Northern Ireland start solids earlier on average than mothers in other countries. A third (34%) of mothers in Northern Ireland have introduced solids by three months compared to 28% of mothers in Scotland and 23% of mothers in England and Wales. Between 1995 and 2000, the decline in the practice of weaning onto solids before 4 months is evident in all countries. In each country, the proportion of mothers who have introduced solids by 3 months has halved over the past five years.

Thus, these results show a definite and ongoing shift towards later introduction of solids. However, a more detailed analysis of the data reveals that a large proportion of mothers were not following the prevailing recommendation –that is for babies to be introduced to solid food at a minimum age of four months, and a maximum of six months. (Although in theory, this should be defined as 17-26 weeks, we discovered that 28% of all mothers recorded that they began their baby on solids at exactly 16 weeks, which many mothers may have interpreted as four months. Therefore we have included these mothers as starting within the "four to six month" window, and this window is defined as 16-26 weeks).

In fact only half (49%) of all mothers began their babies on solids within the timeframe of 16-26 weeks, the large majority of the remainder starting earlier than this (49% of all mothers). A similar pattern emerges in each country, although mothers in Northern Ireland were slightly less likely than mothers in other countries to start solids within the recommended window (43%), and consequently slightly more likely to begin earlier than advised (55%).

Thus the figures indicate that although, over time, there has been an ongoing movement towards later introduction of solids, a very high proportion of mothers are still starting solid food earlier than is generally thought desirable.

Table 9.1, Figure 9.1

Table 9.1

Age of introduction of solid food by country (1995 and 2000 United Kingdom)

	England & Wales		Scotland		Northern Ireland		United Kingdom	
	1995	2000	1995	2000	1995	2000	1995	2000
	Percentage giving solid food							
6 weeks	7	3	8	4	8	3	7	3
8 weeks	12	4	22	7	18	8	13	5
3 months (13 weeks)	54	23	64	28	63	34	56	24
4 months (17 weeks)	91	85	91	83	92	85	91	85
6 months (26 weeks)	99	98	99	99	100	98	99	98
9 months (39 weeks)*	100	100	100	100	100	100	100	100
Before 16 weeks		47		50		55		49
Between 16 & 26 weeks†Δ		51		49		43		49
After 26 weeks†		2		1		2		2
Bases (Stage 3 mothers)	4569	4112	1856	1718	1464	1437	5160	7267

*Based on a reduced number of cases excluding those babies who had not reached this age by Stage 3
† Data not available for 1995
Δ See third paragraph of section 9.1.1, page 164 for an explanation of the derivation of this scale

Figure 9.1

Age at introduction of solids by country (United Kingdom (2000)

Base: All Stage 3 mothers

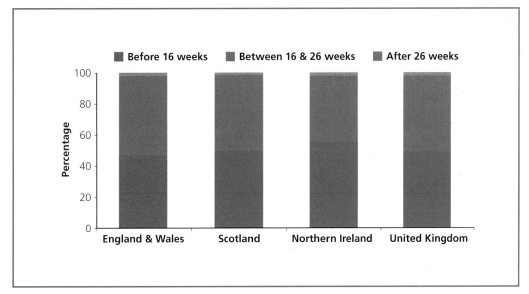

9.1.2   Variation in the age of introduction of solids

Feeding method (breast or infant formula)

Table 9.2 analyses the age of introduction of solids by whether the mother was breastfeeding at the stage of survey when she said she introduced solids. It is not possible to tell from the survey what the mothers' method of feeding was at the time she introduced solids. Therefore this data should be taken as an indication of a relationship between feeding method and introduction of solids, rather than a precise association.

As in previous years, mothers of babies who were not breastfed were more likely to give solid foods earlier. Among mothers who were bottle feeding exclusively, 3% had introduced solid foods by six weeks, and 28% by 3 months, compared with 1% and 12% respectively of mothers who were giving milk only from the breast at the time of weaning. Mothers who fed both breast and bottle milk at the time of weaning fell between these two sets of results.

Table 9.2

Table 9.2
Age at introduction of solid food, by method of feeding at relevant stage (United Kingdom 2000)*

	Breastfed	Breastfed & bottlefed	Not breastfed	All babies†
		Percentage giving solid food		
6 weeks	1	2	3	3
8 weeks	1	3	6	5
3 months (13 weeks)	12	16	28	24
4 months (17 weeks)	79	83	88	85
6 months (26 weeks)	98	99	99	98
9 months (39 weeks)**	100	100	100	100
Base (All Stage 3 mothers)	*986*	*888*	*5284*	*7267*

* See text for an explanation of how this table has been derived
**Based on a reduced number of cases excluding those babies who had not reached this age by Wave 3
† Includes some cases where feeding method at relevant stage not known

Birth order

There is no difference in the pattern of age of starting solid foods by birth order. Mothers of first babies were as likely to have introduced solids by 3 months as mothers of later babies (both 24%).   They were also equally likely to have begun solids within the recommended 16 to 26 week window (around half of all mothers in each group doing so).

Table 9.3

Solid foods

Table 9.3
Age at introduction of solid food, by birth order (United Kingdom 2000)

	First births	Later births	All births
	Percentage giving solid food		
6 weeks	2	3	3
8 weeks	4	5	5
3 months (13 weeks)	24	24	24
4 months (17 weeks)	87	83	85
6 months (26 weeks)	98	98	98
9 months (39 weeks)*	100	100	100
Before 16 weeks	49	46	49
Between 16 & 26 weeksΔ	49	52	49
After 26 weeks	2	2	2
Base (Stage 3 mothers)	3367	3900	7267

Δ See third paragraph of section 9.1.1, page 164 for an explanation of the derivation of this scale

Baby's birthweight

In investigating which babies are introduced to solids at an earlier age, it is not possible to look directly at whether bigger babies who may have a more demanding appetite are introduced to solids any earlier than smaller babies, since no information was collected on the weight or length of the baby at the time the questionnaires were completed. However, as babies growing normally will do so at a rate related to their birthweight, this can be used as an indicator of weight in later infancy.

The pattern was similar to that found in previous years, with mothers of higher birthweight babies tending to introduce solid food at an earlier age. For example, one in four (26%) mothers of babies weighing 3,500 grammes or more at birth had introduced solid foods by three months, compared with one in seven (14%) mothers whose babies weighed under 2,500 grammes. Among this lowest birthweight group, only three-quarters (73%) had introduced solids by four months, compared with over eight in ten in the other birthweight categories. Mothers of babies in this lowest birthweight group were consequently more likely to have followed recommended guidelines with three-fifths (62%) starting within the 16-26 week time-frame compared to a little under half (46%) of mothers of babies in the highest birthweight group.

Table 9.4, Figure 9.2

Table 9.4

Age at introduction of solid food, by birthweight (United Kingdom, 2000)

| | Birthweight of baby | | | | All |
	< 2500g	2500-2999g	3000-3499g	3500 +	babies**
	Percentage giving solid food				
6 weeks	1	2	3	3	3
8 weeks	1	4	6	5	5
3 months (13 weeks)	14	22	23	26	24
4 months (17 weeks)	73	84	87	87	85
6 months (26 weeks)	96	99	99	99	98
9 months (39 weeks)*	99	100	100	100	100
Before 16 weeks	34	46	49	53	49
Between 16 & 26 weeksΔ	62	53	50	46	49
After 26 weeks	3	1	1	1	2
Base (All Stage 3 mothers)	*362*	*1101*	*2456*	*3218*	*7267*

*Based on a reduced number of cases excluding those babies who had not reached this age by Wave 3
**Includes some cases where birthweight not known
Δ See third paragraph of section 9.1.1, page 164 for an explanation of the derivation of this scale

Figure 9.2

Age at introduction of solids by baby's birthweight (United Kingdom (2000)

Base: All Stage 3 mothers

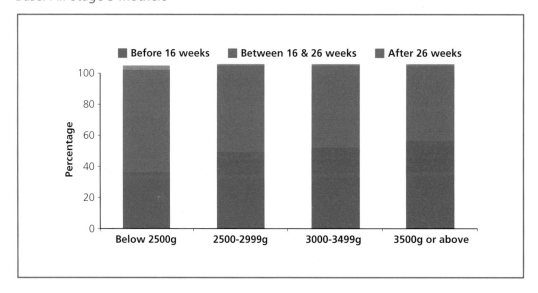

Mother's socio-economic status (NS-SEC)

As might be expected, there was a relationship between socio-economic group and age of introduction of solids. Mothers classified to the highest occupational group were less likely to have introduced solids by three months (17%) compared to mothers in the lowest occupational category (29%) or who had never worked (31%).

However, two-fifths (42%) of higher occupation mothers still introduced solids earlier than recommended, which compares to around a half in each of the other occupational groups.

Table 9.5, Figure 9.3

Table 9.5
Age at introduction of solid food, by mother's socio-economic group (NS-SEC) (United Kingdom, 2000)

	Higher occupations	Intermediate occupations	Lower occupations	Never worked	Unclassi-fied
	Percentage giving solid food				
6 weeks	2	2	4	5	2
8 weeks	3	4	7	7	5
3 months (13 weeks)	17	22	29	31	27
4 months (17 weeks)	84	86	87	82	83
6 months (26 weeks)	98	98	98	95	97
9 months (39 weeks)*	100	100	100	100	100
Before 16 weeks	42	48	51	50	42
Between 16 & 26 weeksΔ	56	50	47	45	55
After 26 weeks	2	2	2	5	3
*Base (All Stage 3 mothers)***	*2315*	*1558*	*1982*	*769*	*644*

*Based on a reduced number of cases excluding those babies who had not reached this age by Stage 3
Δ See third paragraph of section 9.1.1, page 164 for an explanation of the derivation of this scale

Figure 9.3
Age at introduction of solids by mother's socio-economic group (United Kingdom (2000)

Base: All Stage 3 mothers

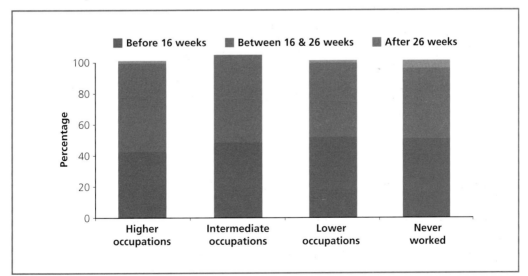

Social class based on occupation of husband or partner

In order to allow comparisons with 1995, the data on age of introduction of solids have also been analysed by partner's social class. The later introduction of solids in 2000 as compared to 1995 is evident within all social class groups, with mothers in 2000 being two to two-and-a-half times less likely than in 1995 to have introduced solids by 3 months within each category. The largest proportional shifts were seen in social class groups II (from 45% to 17% giving solids at 3 months) and IIINM (from 54% to 21%).

Table 9.6

Table 9.6
Age of introduction of solid food based on current or last occupation of husband or partner (Great Britain 1995,United Kingdom, 2000)*

	I		II		IIINM		IIIM		IV		V		No partner/ Unclassified	
	1995	2000	1995	2000	1995	2000	1995	2000	1995	2000	1995	2000	1995	2000
						Percentage giving solid food								
6 weeks	2	1	4	2	5	2	7	3	8	4	9	5	12	4
8 weeks	3	2	7	2	10	4	14	5	13	8	19	8	22	7
3 months	35	16	45	17	54	21	59	27	58	28	68	35	67	28
4 months	88	79	88	82	91	87	93	88	92	87	94	85	93	85
6 months	98	99	100	98	100	98	99	98	100	98	99	97	99	97
9 months **	100	100	100	100	100	100	100	100	100	100	100	100	100	100
Base (All Stage 3 mothers)	*341*	*539*	*1296*	*1900*	*390*	*663*	*1237*	*1946*	*537*	*774*	*180*	*286*	*1017*	*1161*

*Note that 1995 data is based on Great Britain
* *Based on a reduced number of cases excluding babies who had not reached this age at Stage 3

Age left full-time education

Table 9.7 displays the age of introduction of solid food by educational level. Mothers completing their education below the age of 17 introduced solids earlier on average than more educated mothers. Three in ten mothers (29%) in the lowest educational group had introduced solids before 4 months, compared with only one in six mothers (17%) in the highest educational group.

There was also a wide variation by educational level in the proportion of mothers introducing solids within the recommended window. Three-fifths of mothers (60%) in the highest educational group had begun solids within the 16-26 weeks window, compared with only 45% of mothers in the lowest educational group. In fact, a little over half of mothers educated to age 16 or under (53%) were introducing solids before the recommended age.

Table 9.7

Table 9.7

Age at introduction of solid food, by age left full-time education (United Kingdom, 2000)

	16 or under	17 or 18	19+	All mothers**
	%	%	%	%
2 weeks	*	*	*	*
6 weeks	4	2	1	3
8 weeks	7	4	3	5
3 months (13 weeks)	29	24	17	24
4 months (17 weeks)	87	86	81	85
6 months (26 weeks)	98	98	97	98
9 months (39 weeks)*	100	100	100	100
Before 16 weeks	53	49	37	49
Between 16 & 26 weeksΔ	45	49	60	49
After 26 weeks	2	2	3	2
Base (All Stage 3 mothers)	2510	2595	2104	7267

*Based on a reduced number of cases excluding those babies who had not reached this age by Stage 3
** Includes some cases where mothers' educational level not known
Δ See third paragraph of section 9.1.1, page 164 for an explanation of the derivation of this scale

Ethnicity

Mothers from ethnic minority backgrounds introduced solids later on average than white mothers. Asian mothers were the least likely to have introduced solids by 3 months, with 14% doing so compared with 25% of white mothers. At four months, Black mothers were the least likely to have introduced solids with 73% having done so compared with 86% of white mothers.

Following on from this, mothers of Asian, Black and mixed ethnic origin were more likely than white mothers to introduce solids within 16-26 weeks. About two in three mothers in each of these groups had introduced solids within the recommended window, compared with only about half of all white mothers. Mothers of Asian, Black and other ethnicity were also more likely than their white counterparts to introduce solids after 6 months (respectively 6%, 6% and 15% compared with 2% of white mothers).

Table 9.8, Figure 9.4

Table 9.8
Age at introduction of solid food, by ethnicity (United Kingdom, 2000)

	White	Asian	Black	Mixed	Other
	%	%	%	%	
6 weeks	3	1	3	2	[7]
8 weeks	5	1	5	3	[7]
3 months (13 weeks)	25	14	17	18	[18]
4 months (17 weeks)	86	80	73	85	[57]
6 months (26 weeks)	98	94	94	97	[85]
9 months (39 weeks)*	100	100	100	100	[100]
Before 16 weeks	48	28	25	36	[30]
Between 16 & 26 weeksΔ	50	66	69	61	[55]
After 26 weeks	2	6	6	3	[15]
Base (All Stage 3 mothers)	*6761*	*149*	*103*	*61*	*[44]*

*Based on a reduced number of cases excluding those babies who had not reached this age by Stage 3
Δ See third paragraph of section 9.1.1, page 164 for an explanation of the derivation of this scale

Figure 9.4
Age at introduction of solids by ethnicity (United Kingdom (2000)
Base: All Stage 3 mothers

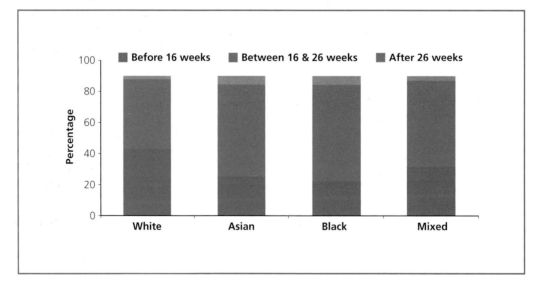

9.2   Solid foods given at different ages

At each stage, mothers who had introduced solids into their babies' diets were asked to list all the cereal, rusks or solid food the baby had eaten on the day before they completed the questionnaire. The mothers were asked to describe each food fully, giving the brand name or saying if it was home-made. For commercial baby food, mothers ticked a column to show whether it was dried or from a tin or a jar. This information was coded from a large range of precodes, which tended to summarise each meal or snack rather than defining each ingredient in the food. Some foods, therefore, may appear to be under-represented as they were eaten as part of a main dish, not coded separately. For example, a home-made meal consisting of chicken, potatoes and carrots would have been coded once as a meat-based meal rather than as three separate codes. The full codeframe can be found in Appendix VI.

Table 9.9 shows what foods were given to babies on the previous day at the different stages, in summarised form. For the small number of mothers who were providing solids at 4-10 weeks, half (51%) had given cereals, most commonly rice cereals (39%). Two in five (38%) had given rusks, and one in eight (13%) had given baby food that was either dried or from a can or a jar. This was twice as likely to be from a can or a jar (9%) than to be dried (4%).

By about four months, the foods given by mothers providing solids were more likely than at stage one to be non-rice cereals, commercially prepared babyfood and home-made food, with a decline in the popularity of rice cereals and rusks. In two thirds (66%) of cases where babies were fed solids, cereals of some type formed part of the diet, with commercial babyfood almost as common an element (62%). Of the commercially-prepared babyfood, food in cans or jars was twice as likely to be provided as dried foods requiring mixing with milk or water before serving (present in 47% and 23% of solid diets respectively).

By Stage 3, when babies were about nine months old the vast majority of mothers (97%) had given solid food the previous day. Four out of five (78%) of these babies had been given cereal; again, as babies grew older they were much more likely to receive non-rice cereals (75% at stage 3) rather than rice cereals (6%). Half (52%) had been given some form of commercially prepared babyfood; almost always this included food from cans or jars (47%), although 9% received dried food. Only one in six (16%) babies on solids at stage 3 still had rusks as part of their diet.

The COMA Report of the Working Group on the Weaning Diet[1] suggests that it is important to give home-prepared foods as part of weaning, in order to introduce the infant to a greater range of flavours and textures than manufactured foods can provide. It is therefore encouraging that seven in ten (70%) mothers providing solid food by stage 3 included home-made food in their baby's diet. The category 'other foods', given by 58% of stage 3 mothers providing solids, covers all types of commercially-prepared adult food.

Table 9.9

Table 9.9

Proportion of mothers who had given different kinds of food on day before completion of questionnaire at each stage of the survey (United Kingdom, 2000)

	4-10 weeks	4-5 months	8-9 months
	Percentage giving each food		
Cereals*	51	66	78
*Rice cereal**	39	27	6
*Other cereal**	17	44	75
Rusk	38	24	16
Commercial babyfood**	13	62	52
*Dried babyfood***	4	23	9
*Babyfood in cans or jars***	9	47	47
*Babyfood, type unspecified***	1	1	*
Home-made food	9	38	70
Other food	2	14	58
Base (All mothers who had given solid food on day before completing questionnaire)	252	7389	7063

Percentages do not add to 100% as some mothers gave more than one answer;
Also, subheadings do not add to headings as some mothers gave more than one answer under each heading
*Baby or adult cereal
**Commercially prepared foods in cans or jars or dried food

The two categories shown in the Table 9.9 labelled "home-made food" and "other food" are broken down in detail in Table 9.10 for stages 2 and 3 (only a small number of stage 1 babies were receiving these types of solids). At about four months, the most popular foods given were vegetables (12% received potatoes, 22% other vegetables) and fresh fruit (19%). One in ten mothers providing solid food gave yoghurt or fromage frais to their baby (11%), and one in twenty (6%) had given their baby a meat-based meal on the day before completing the questionnaire. Compared with 1995, mothers who had given solid food the previous day were slightly more likely to give their four to five month baby yoghurt (11% compared with 5% in 1995) and slightly less likely to be giving meat (6% compared with 10%).

Only 1% of solid diets at stage 2 had included bread or toast on the previous day, but by stage 3 (about nine months) this had risen to a quarter (27%). This reflects the advice given to mothers to avoid gluten (found in cereals such as wheat used in breadmaking) before the infant is six months old, in order to reduce the risk of coeliac disease.

On the day before completion of the stage 3 questionnaire, two in five babies receiving solid foods had eaten yoghurt or fromage frais (43%), a third had had fruit (32%) and one in ten some other dessert (10%). Meat-based meals were the most popular type of combination meal: 36% of babies receiving solids had had a meat-based meal, 9% a fish-based meal and 2% a vegetable-based meal. Overall the results at stage 3 of the questionnaire were broadly similar for 1995 and 2000, although there was a slight decline in the provision of desserts other than fruit and yoghurt (from 17% in 1995 to 10% in 2000) and vegetable-based meals (from 9% to 2%).

Table 9.10

Table 9.10

Proportion of mothers who had introduced solids at Stages 2 and 3 giving different kinds of food on one day (Great Britain 1995, United Kingdom 2000)

Type of food	4-5 months		8-9 months	
	1995* %	2000 %	1995* %	2000 %
Yoghurt	5	11	47	43
Fresh fruit	19	19	34	32
Other dessert	2	1	17	10
Dried fruit or nuts	2	1	1	1
Egg	1	*	4	1
Cheese and dairy produce	2	1	11	10
Meat based meal	10	6	40	36
Fish based meal	2	1	10	9
Vegetable based meal	2	1	9	2
Potatoes	14	12	19	13
Other vegetables	20	22	23	18
Bread/ toast and sandwiches	2	1	35	27
Other foods	2	2	21	20
Base (Mothers giving solid food on day before completing questionnaire)	*4898*	*7389*	*5060*	*7063*

Percentages do not add to 100% as some mothers gave more than one answer
* Note that 1995 data is based on Great Britain

In the stage three questionnaire, mothers were asked how often they gave their baby different types of foods. The results are presented in Table 9.11, which also presents results for 1995 on the same measures. The very small proportion of mothers who had not introduced their baby to solids by stage three are included in the 'Never' categories. The majority of stage three mothers in 2000 gave their baby some food containing carbohydrates at least once a day: four out of five (82%) gave cereals or rusk, almost half gave bread (45%) and one in five (19%) rice or pasta. Seven out of ten (70%) gave dairy products every day, a considerable increase on the level seen in 1995 (55%). About half gave cooked vegetables (53%) and puddings or desserts (49%) every day.

The majority of mothers gave most of the different food types at least once a week. The exceptions to this were raw vegetables, eggs, and sweets and chocolates – in each of these cases the majority of mothers gave them to their babies less than once a week or never. In particular, 44% never gave their baby raw vegetables and 42% never gave eggs (although mothers were less likely to avoid each of these food types than in 1995), and 33% never gave sweets or chocolates to their babies. Foods which are avoided, and the reasons why, will be looked at in more detail in Section 9.3.

Table 9.11

Table 9.11

Frequency with which mothers gave different types of food at stage 3 (Great Britain 1995, United Kingdom 2000)

	1995*	2000		1995*	2000
	%	%		%	%
Cereal or rusk			**Raw vegetables**		
At least once a day	86	82	At least once a day	5	6
At least once a week	10	11	At least once a week	21	25
Less than once a week	2	2	Less than once a week	18	17
Never	2	3	Never	57	44
Rice or pasta			**Cooked vegetables**		
At least once a day	12	19	At least once a day	47	53
At least once a week	63	62	At least once a week	47	39
Less than once a week	12	7	Less than once a week	3	2
Never	13	7	Never	5	3
Bread			**Raw fruit**		
At least once a day	46	45	At least once a day	30	37
At least once a week	36	36	At least once a week	42	40
Less than once a week	8	6	Less than once a week	11	8
Never	11	8	Never	17	10
Meat			**Cooked fruit**		
At least once a day	29	35	At least once a day	15	17
At least once a week	51	47	At least once a week	39	38
Less than once a week	7	5	Less than once a week	18	16
Never	14	9	Never	28	23
Fish			**Cheese, yoghurt, fromage frais**		
At least once a day	4	4	At least once a day	55	70
At least once a week	51	51	At least once a week	34	23
Less than once a week	21	18	Less than once a week	5	2
Never	25	20	Never	6	4
Eggs			**Puddings or desserts**		
At least once a day	2	1	At least once a day	49	49
At least once a week	26	25	At least once a week	32	28
Less than once a week	26	24	Less than once a week	10	10
Never	47	42	Never	9	9
Potatoes			**Sweets or chocolate**		
At least once a day	31	31	At least once a day	7	8
At least once a week	60	60	At least once a week	33	31
Less than once a week	5	3	Less than once a week	28	25
Never	4	3	Never	32	33
Peas, beans, lentils, Chickpeas					
At least once a day	12	15			
At least once a week	54	54			
Less than once a week	14	12			
Never	19	13			
Base (All Stage 3 mothers)	*5180*	*7267*	*Base (All Stage 3 mothers)*	*5180*	*7267*

* Note that 1995 data is based on Great Britain

Table 9.12 shows the how the frequency of giving different types of food varies by mother's socio-economic group. Mothers from higher socio-economic groups were more likely than mothers in lower groups or who had never worked to give rice or pasta, meat, fish, cooked vegetables, fruit (raw and cooked), and dairy products with a frequency of at least three times a week. On the other hand, mothers in lower occupations or who had never worked were more likely than those in higher occupations to give their babies on a regular basis eggs and puddings or desserts. They were also considerably more likely to give sweets or chocolates with this frequency; mothers who had never worked were around three times more likely to give sweets or chocolates at least three times a week (29%) than mothers in higher occupations (11%).

Table 9.12

Table 9.12

Percentage giving different foods at least three times a week at Stage 3 by mother's socio-economic group (NS-SEC) (United Kingdom, 2000)

	Higher occupations	Intermediate occupations	Lower occupations	Never worked	Unclassi-fied
	Percentage giving at least three times a week				
Cereal or rusks	92	88	88	85	85
Rice or pasta	60	53	44	41	56
Bread	68	66	66	66	68
Meat	74	69	65	51	66
Fish	25	22	21	15	22
Eggs	6	5	8	11	8
Potatoes	75	74	74	72	72
Peas, beans, pulses	42	44	47	47	47
Raw vegetables	18	16	18	17	19
Cooked vegetables	90	82	78	66	79
Raw fruit	68	63	57	53	65
Cooked fruit	53	36	30	22	33
Cheese, yoghurt etc.	90	88	89	80	81
Puddings or desserts	60	65	71	69	64
Sweets or chocolate	11	16	23	29	22
Base (All Stage 3 mothers)	*2315*	*1558*	*1982*	*769*	*644*

Consumption of meat

Meat and meat products are rich in haem iron which can be readily absorbed by infants. The Department of Health therefore recommends that foods containing haem iron should be introduced by six to eight months[1]. In order to focus further on consumption of meat at stage three when the babies were about nine months old, mothers were asked whether their baby had ever had meat, how often they gave meat, and, of those who did not give meat, why they were not doing so.

Compared with 1995, mothers in 2000 were giving meat more frequently at stage three of the survey. As shown in Table 9.11 earlier, a third (35%) gave meat every day in 2000, compared with 29% in 1995, with a corresponding fall in the number who never gave meat nowadays – 14% in 1995, 9% in 2000.

Among babies at Stage 3 who had been introduced to solids, around a third (35%) had been given meat on a daily basis, and three-quarters (73%) were fed meat at least three times a week (77%). This is very similar to the frequency seen in 1995. As in previous years, there were variations in the frequency of eating meat by social class. Table 9.13 displays the results by social class based on husband and partner for 1995 and 2000, so that trends over time can be surmised. There is a general trend for increased daily consumption of meat across most social class groups, although significant increases can only be observed in groups II, IIINM, IIIM and no partner/unclassified.

Table 9.13

Table 9.13
Frequency of consumption of meat at stage 3, by social class as defined by current or last occupation of husband or partner (Great Britain 1995,United Kingdom 2000)*

	I		II		IIINM		IIIM		IV		V		No partner/ Unclassified	
	1995 %	2000 %	1995 %	2000 %	1995 %	2000 %	1995 %	2000 %	1995 %	2000 %	1995 %	2000 %	1995 %	2000 %
Every day	34	35	31	36	29	35	29	37	31	36	29	31	26	33
At least 3 times a week	73	73	69	72	71	71	67	69	67	66	66	60	61	60
Ever	91	94	94	93	94	93	93	93	92	93	95	92	90	90
Base (All Stage 3 mothers who had ever given their baby solids)	337	539	1296	1879	389	660	1233	1912	535	765	177	281	1014	1144

Mothers who had not given their baby meat at all were asked why, and the reasons given are shown in Table 9.14 (the first three answers were listed as options in the questionnaire, the remaining two specified answers were coded from spontaneously given answers. Three out of five mothers not feeding meat (60%) said that their baby was not ready for it yet, whilst three in ten (29%) said they intended to give their baby a vegetarian diet. These two answers accounted for the vast majority of cases. Only a small proportion (4%) said it was because their baby did not like meat. Compared with 1995, there has been a significant drop in the proportion of people mentioning media health scares, which relates to the much higher profile of BSE/CJD at the time of the previous wave.

Table 9.14

The COMA Report of the Working Group on the Weaning Diet[1] states that it is important for babies having vegetarian diets to be provided with high levels of vitamin C, as this enhances the absorption of iron present in non-meat sources of iron. One method of ensuring this is by giving supplements of vitamin C. However, only one in five (21%) of babies who did not have meat in their diets were receiving extra vitamins (either directly, or through breastfeeding at stage 3 by mothers who took vitamin supplements at the time). This remains unchanged from the corresponding proportion in 1995 (20%).

Table 9.14
Reasons for not offering meat (Great Britain 1995, United Kingdom, 2000)*

	1995	2000
	%	%
Baby does not like meat	8	4
Baby is not ready to eat meat	51	60
Baby given a vegetarian diet	31	29
Media scares/ publicity (incl. BSE/FMD)	8	1
Other reasons	2	2
Base (Stage 3 mothers who had never given their baby meat)	*369*	*446*
* Note that 1995 data is based on Great Britain		

Giving drinks containing vitamin C

The COMA Report also suggests that vitamin C enriched fruit drinks consumed with a meal may be useful to aid the absorption of iron from a meal. As shown in table 9.15, at stage two, when the babies were aged about four months, two in five (37%) mothers in the United Kingdom who gave their baby solids gave a drink containing vitamin C at the same meal. Results were broadly similar by country.

Compared with 1995, there has been a drop in the proportion of mothers giving vitamin C drinks to their four-month-old babies who had begun on solids; in 1995 the level was 47%. Similar shifts are also evident in each country. This tallies with the findings reported in Chapter 8 which showed a general reduction in the provision of drinks such as fruit juice, with more mothers giving plain water instead.

Table 9.15

Table 9.15
Proportion of mothers who gave drinks containing vitamin C with solids at stage 2, by country (1995 and 2000)

	England & Wales		Scotland		Northern Ireland		United Kingdom	
	1995 %	2000 %	1995 %	2000 %	1995 %	2000 %	1995 %	2000 %
Yes, usually	21	17	23	18	24	19	21	17
Yes, sometimes	26	20	28	23	26	21	26	20
No, never	53	63	50	59	50	60	53	62
Base (Stage 2 mothers who gave their babies solid food at stage 2)								
	4431	*4336*	*1827*	*1884*	*1444*	*1441*	*5002*	*7624*

Using milk to mix food

Mothers who had introduced solid foods were asked if they used milk to mix up their babies' food and, if so, which type of milk they used. At each of stages two and three, seven out of ten mothers had used milk to mix up food (71% at stage two, 69% at stage three).

At stage two, when the babies were around four months old, the majority of mothers using milk to mix food used infant formula milk (89%). One in twenty (6%) used expressed breastmilk, with only a small proportion using cow's milk (3%) or some other type of milk (2%). By stage three, when babies were around nine months old, cow's milk was used in two-thirds (69%) of cases where milk was used, with a quarter (27%) using infant formula milk and one in five (22%) follow-on formula milk.

Compared with 1995, fewer mothers at either stage used cow's milk to mix their babies' food – at that time 8% at stage two and 74% at stage three of those using milk used cow's milk when mixing food. Follow-on formula milk was more commonly used at stage three in 2000 than in 1995 (22% compared with 17%).

Mothers in Northern Ireland who used milk to mix baby food were more likely than those in other countries to use cow's milk at both stages: 7% at stage two, and 75% at stage three (compared with 3% and 69% of other mothers respectively). They were also less likely to use follow-on formula milk at stage three (13% compared with 22% of mothers in other countries using milk to mix food).

Table 9.16

Although 27% of breastfeeding mothers who used milk to mix solid foods used expressed breast milk at stage two to do so, nearly two thirds (63%) used infant formula milk. Similarly, at stage three only 9% of breastfeeding mothers mixing solids with milk used breast milk. The majority used cow's milk (67%), but infant formula and follow-on formula milk were also both more commonly used than breastmilk.

Table 9.17

9.3   Influences on the choice of solid food

In the stage two questionnaire, mothers who gave solids to their babies were asked what influenced their decision on what type of solid food to give. This was an open question without any prompting or precoding, and many mothers mentioned more than one factor – although one in ten (11%) did not answer this question. Table 9.18 shows the answers grouped as being related to nutritional and dietary factors, or other factors related to the mother or baby. Only answers given by at least 5% of mothers in the base are recorded.

Table 9.16
Type of milk used to mix up food at stages 2 and 3, by country (2000)

	England & Wales	Scotland	Northern Ireland	United Kingdom
	%	%	%	%
4-5 months:				
Cow's milk	3	4	7	3
Infant formula milk	89	88	90	89
Expressed breast milk	6	8	4	6
Something else	2	2	2	2
Base (Stage 2 mothers who used milk to mix up their babies' food)	*3088*	*1268*	*994*	*5399*
8-9 months:				
Cow's milk	69	71	75	69
Infant formula milk	27	26	25	27
Follow-on formula milk	23	21	13	22
Expressed breast milk	3	4	1	3
Something else	2	2	2	2
Base (Stage 3 mothers who used milk to mix up their babies' food)	*2796*	*1218*	*1015*	*4942*

Percentages do not add up to 100% as some mothers gave more than one answer

Table 9.17
Type of milk used to mix up food at stages 2 and 3, by feeding method (United Kingdom, 2000)

	Breastfeeding*	Not breastfeeding	All mothers
	%	%	%
4-5 months:			
Cow's milk	4	4	3
Infant formula milk	63	96	89
Expressed breast milk	27	*	6
Something else	2	2	2
Base (Stage 2 mothers who used milk to mix up babies' food)	*1210*	*4123*	*5399*
8-9 months:			
Cow's milk	67	69	69
Infant formula milk	18	28	27
Follow-on formula milk	26	21	22
Expressed breast milk	9	2	3
Something else	4	2	2
Base (Stage 3 mothers who used milk to mix up babies' food)	*760*	*4176*	*4942*

Percentages do not add up to 100% as some mothers gave more than one answer
*Includes mothers who breastfed and gave manufactured baby milk

One in four (26%) referred to nutritional value of the food in general terms. However, some mothers were more specific, the most common mentions being sugar content (17%), vitamins (12%), gluten (11%) and salt (10%). In terms of dietary factors more generally, one in six (13%) mentioned the importance of fresh fruit or vegetables in their babies' diet, and one in ten (9%) mentioned organic produce.

Of the non-nutritional factors, most were related to the baby's rather than the mother's needs. Variety of flavours was in fact the most commonly mentioned factor of all for stage two mothers, with 29% giving this answer. Variety of textures was mentioned by 5%, with 31% giving at least one of these two answers. The next most common non-nutritional factor was baby's preferences, mentioned by one in six (16%). One in ten said it was important to have foods that were right for the baby's age (12%), and a similar proportion saying they chose foods with good flavour (10%).

At the stage three questionnaire, mothers who gave solids were asked if they avoided giving their baby foods that contained particular ingredients, and if so which and why. Mothers recorded the ingredients and reasons, and the answers were coded. Half (47%) of stage three mothers across the United Kingdom who had begun their baby on solids said they avoided particular ingredients. This is similar to the level seen in 1990 (51%), after an increase in 1995 when 59% of British mothers said they avoided ingredients (comparable figure for 2000 is still 47% when restricted to Great Britain only).

Table 9.18

Table 9.18
What mothers took into account when deciding what solid foods to give at stage 2 (United Kingdom 2000)

Nutritional factors:	Proportion mentioning %	Factors related to baby:	Proportion mentioning %
Nutritional value (general)	26	Variety of flavours	29
Sugar content	17	Baby's preferences	16
Vitamin content	12	Baby's age	12
Gluten content	11	Flavour/ not too bland	10
Salt content	10	Consistency	7
Additives	8	Baby's appetite	7
Mineral content (not salt)	5	Variety of textures	5
		Number of meals a day	5
Other dietary factors:			
Fresh fruit/ vegetables	13	**Factors related to mothers:**	
Organic/ home-grown	9	Ease of preparation	7
Prefer home-made food	8	What family is eating	5
		Brand name	5
		Advice received	5
Base (Stage 2 mothers giving solids)	7624	*Base (Stage 2 mothers giving solids)*	7624

Percentages do not add up to 100% as some mothers gave more than one answer

This trend is linked to the high profile of BSE at the time of the 1995 survey, when avoidance of beef was relatively common. In 1995, of all mothers avoiding ingredients in their babies' diet at about eight months, two-fifths (40%) avoided beef compared with only one in twenty (5%) in 2000.

Table 9.19

Table 9.19
Ingredients avoided by mothers who gave solid food at stage 3 (Great Britain 1995, United Kingdom, 2000)*

	1995	2000
	%	%
Added ingredients:		
Sugar	40	33
Salt	25	33
Additives	9	8
Colourings	4	3
Preservatives	2	2
Fat	4	1
Flavourings	-	1
Other additives	2	2
Specific foodstuffs:		
Nuts	14	30
Eggs	12	15
Beef	40	5
Spices	7	2
Dairy produce generally		9
Meat generally		8
Honey		6
Seafood/ fish	37**	5
Gluten/ wheat		5
Particular fruits or vegetables		5
Sweets/ chocolate		2
Other specific foodstuffs		4
Base (Mothers at stage 3 avoiding certain ingredients)	*2940*	*3385*

Percentages do not add up to 100% as some mothers gave more than one answer
* Note that 1995 results based on Great Britain
** Responses not available separately for 1995

The other types of ingredients avoided are presented in Table 9.20 for the two survey years. Sugar and salt were the most commonly avoided ingredients (both ingredients avoided by 33% of all mothers), followed by nuts (30%) and eggs (15%). Compared with 1995, the proportions of mothers avoiding salt and nuts has increased (from 25% to 33% and from 14% to 30% respectively). The latter finding is likely to be related to the higher profile of nut allergies over recent years.

Mothers who avoided foods were asked their reasons for this. The most common reason given for avoiding particular ingredients was concern about food allergies, mentioned in a third of all cases of avoidance (35%). This has risen in recent years, and in particular has doubled since 1990, from around one in twelve mothers who gave solids in the 1990 survey (based on mothers in Great Britain). One in four (26%) of those avoiding ingredients gave a general answer about it not being beneficial, and one in five (20%) a general answer about it being harmful. A further one in five (18%) said the ingredients they avoided were bad for the teeth, and one in ten (10%) said it was because of media publicity.

Table 9.20

Table 9.20

Reasons for avoiding particular ingredients at stage 3 (Great Britain 1995, United Kingdom, 2000)*

	1995	2000
	%	%
Allergies	26	35
Not beneficial	44	26
Harmful	20	20
Bad for teeth	25	18
Media publicity/ scares	42	10
On advice†		7
Avoid sweet tooth	5	6
Digestion problems†		5
Hyperactivity	4	2
Other reasons relevant to diet†		8
Other reasons not relevant to diet†		8
Base (Mothers at stage 3 avoiding certain ingredients)	*2873*	*3385*

Percentages do not add up to 100% as some mothers gave more than one answer
* Note that 1995 results based on Great Britain
† Data not available for 1995

9.4 Difficulties with weaning

The COMA Report[1] recommends that 'by the age of one year the diet should be mixed and varied'. Mothers who gave solid food to their baby were asked in the stage three questionnaire to describe the variety of food their baby (then aged about eight to nine months) generally ate, using a set of precoded answers. Two thirds (68%) said that their baby ate most things, and only one in twenty (5%) described their baby as a fussy eater.

Mothers in higher occupations were more likely to describe their baby as eating a greater variety of foods compared with mothers who had never worked (72% compared with 61%), and were consequently less likely to describe their baby as a fussy eater (3% compared to 9%).

Table 9.21

Table 9.21

Variety of solid food baby generally eats at stage 3, by mother's socio-economic group (NS-SEC) (United Kingdom, 2000)

	Higher occupations	Intermediate occupations	Lower occupations	Never worked	Unclassi-fied	All mothers
	%	%				
Eats most things	72	66	68	61	69	68
Eats a reasonable variety of things	25	29	26	30	25	26
Fussy or faddy eater	3	4	6	9	5	5
Base (Babies given solids at Stage 3)	*2297*	*1544*	*1957*	*750*	*631*	*7180*

When their babies were about nine months old, mothers who had introduced solid foods were asked if they had found it difficult weaning their baby onto solids. One in ten (10%) had experienced difficulties, a proportion that did not vary significantly between the constituent countries of the United Kingdom (10% in England and Wales and Scotland, 9% in Northern Ireland).

Mothers whose baby had been born at a low birthweight (under 2500g) were slightly more likely than those whose babies were born at 3500g or over to have had difficulties weaning (14% compared to 9%). Mothers of ethnic minority backgrounds were considerably more likely to have had problems weaning their baby onto solids. In particular, a quarter (25%) of Black mothers and a fifth (21%) of Asian mothers reported problems compared with 9% of white mothers. However, these two trends will be related as Black, Asian and mothers from other ethnic backgrounds had babies of lower average birthweights when compared with white mothers.

Table 9.22

Mothers who had encountered difficulties with weaning onto solids were asked what type of problems they had faced, by presenting a set of precoded answers. The most frequently cited problem in this group was that the baby would only take a limited range of foods (52% of mothers who had found weaning difficult). Other difficulties were baby refusing all solids (24%), preferring drinks to food (22%), being disinterested in food (22%), and vomiting (18%).

Table 9.23

Table 9.22

Proportion of mothers who had found it difficult weaning their baby onto solid food by baby's birthweight and ethnicity (United Kingdom, 2000)

	Proportion reporting difficulties	Base (Stage 3 mothers whose babies had been given solid food
Baby's birthweight		
Less than 2500g	14	379
2500-2999g	11	1044
3000-3499g	10	2380
3500+	9	3338
Mother's ethnic group		
White	9	6774
Asian	21	105
Black	25	71
Mixed/Other**	15	84
All mothers*	10	7180

* Includes some mothers for whom ethnicity and/or birthweight not recorded
** These categories combined due to small base sizes

Table 9.23

Difficulties with weaning reported by mothers at stage 3 (United Kingdom 2000)

	%
Baby would only take certain solids	52
Baby would not take solids	24
Baby prefers drinks to food	22
Baby was disinterested in food	22
Baby vomiting	18
Some other reason	6
No answer given	3
Base (Mothers giving solid food at stage 3 who found it difficult to wean their baby)	727

Percentages do not add up to 100% as some mothers gave more than one answer

[1]   Department of Health. Weaning and the Weaning Diet, Report of the Working Group on the Weaning Diet of the Committee on Medical Aspects of Food Policy. HMSO (London: 1994)

[2]   For results before 1995, see Foster K, Lader D, Cheeseborough S Infant Feeding 1995, HMSO (London, 1997)

Appendix I
Survey Methodology

I.1   Sample design

The sample design for the Infant Feeding Survey in 2000 replicated the design from 1995 and previous years. In order to obtain a sufficiently large sample in Northern Ireland and Scotland, births in these countries were given a greater chance of selection than in England and Wales. The aim was to achieve sample sizes as obtained in 1995, and detailed below.

England & Wales	5200
Scotland	2150
Northern Ireland	1750
United Kingdom	9100

The 2000 survey continued the practice, established in 1985, of over-sampling births to mothers in the following social class categories:

- social class V (as defined by current or last occupation of husband or partner)
- mothers who didn't register a partner on the birth certificate
- mothers whose social class could not be classified, either because of inadequate information about the husband or partner's job or because he had never worked

Previous surveys have shown a strong association between social class and infant feeding practices and over-sampling ensures that there are sufficient numbers for analysis as a separate group if necessary. Births to women in these categories were given twice the chance of selection of other births.

I.2   Drawing the sample in each country

The samples in each country were selected from births occurring in a given range of dates between August and October 2000 and were designed to be representative of all births in these periods. The number of days chosen varied between countries, and depended on the estimated number of births in each social class group which would be registered within the sampling period and other details of the sampling scheme in each country. The time periods were almost identical to those used in 1995, and are listed below.

England & Wales	August 19th to September 26th
Scotland	August 19th to September 6th classes I-IV
	August 19th to September 22nd other births*
Northern Ireland	August 12th to 19th October

* Due to administrative difficulties, the sampling was slightly different in Scotland than in other countries in 2000. This was not the original intention, however it ensured the correct sample profile was maintained and does not affect the consistency of the findings between countries.

The sampling frame in each country consisted of all registrations for births on the selected dates that were received by the appropriate registration office[1] within a specified sampling period up to a maximum of eight weeks after the birth.

England and Wales

A two-stage design was used in England and Wales. The 100 first-stage units were a sample of registration sub-districts or groups of smaller sub-districts. As far as possible these were the same sub-districts as used on the previous Infant Feeding Surveys. The original sub-districts used in the first survey in 1975 were selected with probability proportional to the number of births. At each subsequent survey, variation in birth rates necessitated some change to the selected sub-districts. The criteria used to determine which districts were dropped and which districts replaced them is called the Keyfitz procedure[2]. This method aims to ensure a probability of selection of each sub-district that reflects changes in birth rates while minimising the number of sampling units that need to be changed.

The registration districts selected are listed in Appendix IV.

The 100 birth registration sub-districts selected for the sample record varying amount of births and in total too many births for inclusion in the sample. Consequently a randomly selected proportion of births (varying according to the anticipated number of births in each birth district) were selected on an ongoing basis during the birth period; these were then coded with social class classifications.

All births to fathers of Social class V, father not known and not classified were then part of sample along with one in two births to Social Class I-IV. This produced a total of 7382 births in England and Wales.

Scotland

In Scotland a similar sampling approach was taken to that used in England and Wales. However, because there are fewer births in these countries the birth period was chosen so that all births to mothers in Social class V, those with no partner or mothers whose social class could not be classified were selected, and one in two of all other births was then selected. This yielded 3113 births in Scotland.

Northern Ireland

The intention was that the sample in Northern Ireland would be drawn in the same way as Scotland – i.e. all births to fathers of Social class V, father not known and not classified were to be part of sample along with one in two births to Social Class I-IV. However, the birth rate for the sampled period in Northern Ireland fell slightly below our expectations. Therefore to ensure we met our sample size requirements, we increased the sampling fraction of births to social classes I to IV to three-fifths (59%) of all births rather than one in two (50%). In total, 2617 births were sampled in Northern Ireland

I.3   Questionnaire design

The questionnaires were based on the 1995 versions, although a small number of amendments were. In summary, the following additions and amendments were made:

Stage 1:

Addition of questions about:

- sleeping position of baby
- knowledge of the health advantages of breastfeeding
- whether mothers felt any pressure from health professionals regarding how they should feed their baby
- ethnic background

Smoking module revised to improve the reliability of results and to provide more detail on smoking and pregnancy (see section I.4).

Stage 2:

- New module on childcare and employment plans and how this affected feeding of baby

Stage 3:

- As for Stage 2

In Stages 2 and 3, two versions of the questionnaire were used depending on whether the mother was still breastfeeding at the time of the previous interview. This allowed the questionnaire to be more tailored to mothers' individual circumstances and avoided the use of complex routing.

At Stage 1, in order to test out the new version of the questionnaire, a small-scale pilot was conducted among 10 mothers. Mothers participating in the pilot were recruited from health visitor clinics in London Paddington and Birmingham. Mothers were then asked to complete the questionnaire in the presence of a research executive and any problems regarding the wording or routing were noted. A mixture of breast and bottle-feeding mothers were included in the pilot across a range of social class groups.

At Stage 2, where changes to the questionnaire were less significant, a smaller pilot was conducted among 5 mothers recruited via contacts known to the research team. A similar scale pilot was conducted for Stage 3.

I.4   Note on changes to smoking module

The smoking questions included in the 1995 Infant Feeding Survey were the same as those asked in the 1985 and 1990 surveys. Interest in smoking and pregnancy has increased since 1985 and a review of these questions suggested that they did not indicate respondents' smoking status during pregnancy in sufficient detail.

Prior to 2000, any mother who had smoked cigarettes in the two years before the survey (i.e. about a year before conception) was asked about the average number of cigarettes smoked before, during and after pregnancy. The questions on smoking used in the 2000 Infant Feeding Survey were changed so that the emphasis was on changes in smoking behaviour, rather than simply changes in cigarette consumption. It was felt that the revised questions indicated more reliably mothers' smoking behaviour in pregnancy.

The Tobacco White Paper "Smoking Kills" was published in December 1998 and contains the government's anti-smoking strategy. The White Paper highlighted smoking among pregnant women as a key area, and included the target:

> "*To reduce the percentage of women who smoke during pregnancy from 23% to 15% by the year 2010; with a fall to 18% by the year 2005*".

This target was set using figures from the 1995 Infant Feeding Survey as a baseline. Progress towards the target is being measured using the 2000 survey. However, the changes in the questions on smoking behaviour between the 1995 and 2000 surveys mean that the results from the 2000 survey are not robustly comparable with the 1995 survey. Therefore, progress against the above target can only be estimated from the 2000 figures.

I.5   Fieldwork procedures

Stage 1

For the first stage of fieldwork, the approach to mothers was made through the respective Registration Offices in the different countries. Sampling was conducted by ONS for England & Wales, the GRO in Scotland for the Scottish sample and by NISRA for the Northern Ireland sample. In the case of England, Wales and Scotland, all printing and packing was done by BMRB although ONS handled the despatch as the name and address of the mother could not be released to a survey organisation at this stage. In Northern Ireland, the printing, packing and despatch was carried out exclusively by CSU.

The first questionnaire was sent out during October/November/December 2000 to all mothers included in the initial sample, with the aim of contacting mothers when their babies were between six and ten weeks old (although after a lengthy reminder period, in fact some babies were older than this).

In England, Wales and Scotland, sampling was conducted on a weekly basis and despatch was organised in a staggered fashion such that for each sampling week, questionnaires were aimed to first reach mothers at the time when their baby was approximately 6 weeks old. Although the majority of births were registered within these 6 weeks, an additional 3 sampling weeks were added at the end of fieldwork in order to "mop-up" the late-registered births. This meant that the main despatch took place in 8 phases. An additional mailout phase was also added at the end to account for the extra births sampled in the extended extraction period for Scotland.

In Northern Ireland, the sampling and despatch was phased across 4 birth periods.

The initial mailing included a letter from ONS/GRO/CSU, a pre-serial numbered questionnaire and reply-paid envelope for arrival at BMRB. All outgoing malings were sent first-class with returns costed at second-class. Booking-in of questionnaires was undertaken by BMRB's data capture department.

A blanket reminder was sent out after one week which comprised a reminder letter targeted to all mothers who had not yet responded. A second full-pack reminder was sent out after a further 2 weeks for all those who had still not responded, with a further reminder after an additional 2 weeks. The reminders were sent out in a staggered fashion, following the staggered nature of the sampling and initial despatch. Unlike stages 2 and 3, there was no interviewer follow-up at Stage 1 as names and addresses of non-responding mothers could not be passed to BMRB.

At the end of the wave 1 questionnaire, mothers were asked to give forwarding contact details if they were planning to move and address details were updated in time for the Wave 2 mailout.

The total despatch period lasted between 27 October and 12 January.

Stage 2

Names and addresses of all mothers responding to stages 1 in England, Wales and Scotland were provided by ONS to BMRB. In January 2001, when the babies were approximately four to five months old, a second stage questionnaire was sent to all mothers who had completed the first questionnaire (apart from a small number of mothers who had specifically asked not to be contacted again). BMRB handled the mailout for England, Wales and Scotland while CSU continued to handle the mailout for Northern Ireland.

Mothers who had not replied after two weeks were sent a reminder letter, and mothers still not responding after a further 2 weeks were sent another copy of the questionnaire and a reply-paid envelope. Finally, an attempt was made to obtain a response at the second stage by sending an interviewer to contact mothers who had not replied to the various letters.

Despatch for the postal survey took place in two phases (the second phase including the later respondents to Wave 1). The total despatch period lasted between 9 January and 4 March. The interviewer fieldwork stage covered the period from 5 March to 27 April.

Stage 3

In June 2001, when the babies were approximately eight to nine months old, a third questionnaire was sent to all mothers who had completed the second questionnaire. The fieldwork procedures were the same as at Stage 2. The total despatch period lasted between 4 June and 27 July. The interviewer fieldwork stage covered the period from 30 July to 12 August.

I.6 Response

Response at stage 1

Table I.1 gives details of response by country at Wave 1. Overall, 72% of the original sample of women responded to the first stage questionnaire, this ranging from 68% in Northern Ireland to 74% in England and Wales.

Efforts were made by ONS to identify any baby deaths among the sampled births before sending out the first questionnaire and these cases were removed from the sample before despatch. However, mothers receiving the questionnaire whose baby was no longer with them, for example if the baby had died, been adopted or was in hospital, were not expected to complete a questionnaire but were asked to return the form so that they would not be contacted again. In total, 45 mothers were identified in this category.

There were 53 refusals to participate which included questionnaires returned with an explicit refusal or a refusal via telephone. A further 74 questionnaires were returned blank or incomplete (only the first 2-3 questions answered).

Table I.1

Table I.1
Response rates and non-response at first stage of survey (Oct-Dec 2000)

	England & Wales		Scotland		Northern Ireland		United Kingdom	
	No.	%	No.	%	No.	%	No.	%
Initial sample	7382	100	3113	100	2617	100	13112	100
Total response	**5440**	**74**	**2274**	**73**	**1778**	**68**	**9492**	**72**
Total non-response	**1942**	**26**	**859**	**27**	**839**	**32**	**3620**	**28**
Baby not with mother	33	*	5	*	7	*	45	*
Refusal	33	*	18	1	2	*	53	*
Incomplete questionnaire	48	1	21	1	5	*	74	1
Post returned/not delivered	4	*	4	*	0	0	8	*
No reply	1824	25	811	26	825	32	3440	26

Response at Stage 2

The issued sample at Stage 2 comprised all mothers responding at Stage 1. Response at the second stage of the survey was higher than at the first stage, ranging from 86% in Scotland to 91% in Northern Ireland. The improvement in response rate was largely attributable to the interviewer follow-up of non-respondents. The interviewer follow-up added 17% to response rates overall.

Table I.2

Table I.2
Response rates and non-response at second stage of survey (Jan-March 2001)

	England & Wales		Scotland		Northern Ireland		United Kingdom	
	No.	%	No.	%	No.	%	No.	%
Second stage sample	5440	100	2274	100	1778	100	9492	100
Total response	**4729**	**87**	**1953**	**86**	**1617**	**91**	**8299**	**87**
Due to postal enquiry	3822	70	1592	70	1223	69	6638	70
Due to interviewer contact	907	17	361	16	394	22	1661	17
Total non-response	**711**	**13**	**321**	**14**	**161**	**9**	**1193**	**13**
Not issued - refused at first stage	12	*	7	*	1	*	20	*
Not issued – other reason*	24	*	23	1	0	-	47	*
Baby no longer with mother	10	*	3	*	0	-	13	*
Refusal	35	1	10	*	0	-	45	*
Post returned/not delivered	36	1	20	1	0	-	56	1
Incomplete questionnaire	9	*	2	*	0	*	11	*
No reply from postal stage and interviewer unable to contact	585	11	256	11	160	9	1001	11

* A total of 47 mothers who responded at Stage 1 were excluded from the Stage 2 mailout. This is accounted for by 25 questionnaires returned late at Stage 1, and there was insufficient time for addresses to be obtained from ONS; and 22 cases where we were unable to classify mothers as either a breast or bottle feeder and therefore could not establish which version of the Stage 2 questionnaire should be sent.

Response at Stage 3

The issued sample at Stage 3 comprised all mothers responding at Stage 2. At Stage 3, the total response was 88%. Once again, this high response rate was largely attributable to the interviewer stage which added 14% to the response rate.

Table I.3

Cumulative response rates

Since mothers were only contacted in later stages of the survey if they had responded at the previous one, the effect of non-response at each stage is cumulative. The effective response rate at each stage should therefore be calculated as a proportion of the initial sample. Questionnaires were received at the second stage from 63% of the original sample and this proportion fell to 55% at the third stage.

Table I.4

Table I.3

Response rates and non-response at third stage of survey (June-July 2001)

	England & Wales		Scotland		Northern Ireland		United Kingdom	
	No.	%	No.	%	No.	%	No.	%
Second stage sample	4729	100	1953	100	1617	100	8299	100
Total response	**4112**	**87**	**1718**	**88**	**1437**	**89**	**7267**	**88**
Due to postal enquiry	3563	75	1463	75	1097	68	6123	74
Due to interviewer contact	549	12	255	13	340	21	1144	14
Total non-response	**617**	**13**	**235**	**12**	**180**	**11**	**1032**	**12**
Not issued - refused at second stage	5	*	1	*	4	*	10	*
Baby no longer with mother	5	*	1	*	0	-	6	*
Refusal	16	*	4	*	0	-	20	*
Post returned/not delivered	70	1	42	2	0	-	112	1
Incomplete questionnaire	8	*	10	1	0	-	18	*
No reply from postal stage and interviewer unable to contact	513	11	177	9	176	11	866	10

Table I.4

Summary of response at stages 1, 2 and 3 by country

	England & Wales		Scotland		Northern Ireland		United Kingdom	
	No.	%	No.	%	No.	%	No.	%
Initial sample	7382	100	3113	100	2617	100	13112	100
Response at Stage 1	5440	74	2274	73	1778	68	9492	72
Response at Stage 2	4729	64	1953	63	1617	62	8299	63
Response at Stage 3	4112	56	1718	55	1437	55	7267	55

Comparisons of response rate with 1990 and 1995 survey

Table I.5 shows the response rates for the last three survey years for Stage 1, and for 1995 and 2000 for the later stages. As seen from Table I.5, the response in 2000 at Stage 1 was similar to that obtained in 1995 for England & Wales, and Scotland. In Northern Ireland, the response was slightly lower in 2000 compared with 1995 (68% compared to 72%). Response rates to Stage 1 in 1990 were considerably higher. This is largely explained by the fact that at this time, non-responding mothers were able to be contacted by an interviewer in the field, whereas changes in the data protection regulations did not allow this final follow-up from 1995 onwards. However, postal response was also slightly lower in 1995 and 2000 compared with 1990, and reflects a growing trend for declining response rates to government surveys over the past 10 years or so.

In later stages, the response rates at Stages 2 and 3 in England & Wales and Scotland were similar in 2000 to those obtained in 1995. However, although the overall response rate is similar, there were differences in the proportion of achieved interviews that originated from the postal and interviewer stages. In 1995, in England and Wales, 79% of mothers responding to Stage 1 had responded to Stage 2 by the end of the postal survey, and the interviewer stage picked up only 6% more respondents. However, in 2000, the mothers were less responsive to the postal stage (70% in England and Wales) and the interviewer stage therefore picked up a higher proportion of mothers (17% in England and Wales).

Response in Northern Ireland was slightly lower at all stages in 2000 compared with 1995, resulting in a lower cumulative net response by the end of the three stages (55% compared with 63%).

Table I.5

Table I.5
Response rates at all three stages of the survey, 1990 to 2000

	England & Wales			Scotland			Northern Ireland		
	1990 %	1995 %	2000 %	1990 %	1995 %	2000 %	1990 %	1995 %	2000 %
Stage 1									
Response to postal	80	75	74	76	73	73	75	72	68
Response to interviewer*	9	n/a	n/a	9	n/a	n/a	14	n/a	n/a
Total response rate	89	75	74	85	73	73	90	72	68
Base:	*6467*	*6972*	*7382*	*2597*	*2908*	*3113*	*2041*	*2434*	*2617*
Stage 2									
Response to postal		79	70		79	70		77	69
Response to interviewer		6	17		5	16		17	22
Total response rate		86	87		84	86		94	91
Base:		*5240*	*5440*		*2137*	*2274*		*1753*	*1778*
Stage 3									
Response to postal		82	75		79	75		75	68
Response to interviewer		9	12		9	13		18	12
Total response rate		91	87		89	88		93	89
Base:		*4490*	*4729*		*1798*	*1953*		*1653*	*1617*
Cumulative response									
Initial sample		100	100		100	100		100	100
Response at Stage 1		75	74		73	73		72	68
Response at Stage 2		64	64		62	63		68	62
Response at Stage 3		58	56		55	55		63	55

* Not applicable in 1995 and 2000, as there was no interviewer-administered fieldwork at Stage 1

I.7   Re-weighting the results

Various weights were applied to data from the first and subsequent stages of the survey. These compensated for differences in the probability of selection for mothers in different social class groups and different countries, and for differential non-response at each stage of the survey. The stages of weighting were as follows:

1. *To correct for over-sampling of mothers with partners in Social Class V, whose social class was "other" or unclassifiable or where no partner details were recorded at registration*

    In England, Wales and Scotland, babies born to mothers in the above groups were given twice the chance of selection compared to babies born to mothers whose partner was classified as social class I-IV. Thus babies born to the above categories were given a weight of 0.5.

    In Northern Ireland, the proportion of mothers with a partner classified in social class I-IV sampled was increased to 59% (instead of 50%) compared to 100% of all births in the other categories. This was to correct for a lower-than-anticipated birth count in the sampling period. Thus, all births in Social Class V, other/unclassified and father not present were given a weight of 0.59.

2. *To correct for differential non-response by social class group at the first stage of the survey*

    The overall response rates to the first stage were 74% in England & Wales, 73% in Scotland and 68% in Northern Ireland. Information on social class of mother's partner, based on registration data, was made available for the full sample, including non-respondents. Analysis showed that there was a consistent pattern within each country of declining response through the range from Social Classes I to V (see Table I.6). This was corrected by weighting cases in each social class group within country by the inverse of the response rate for the group.

3. *To correct for over-sampling of births in Scotland and Northern Ireland*

    As births in Scotland and Northern Ireland were given a greater chance of selection than those in England & Wales, they were re-weighted to give the correct balance when showing results for the United Kingdom. The weights were derived by comparing the proportion of sampled births in each country with the proportion of all births in 2000 for the sampling periods in each country3. The resulting weighting factors were 0.189 for births in Scotland and 0.173 in NI (and 1.00 in England & Wales).

4. *To correct for differential response by initial feeding method and by country at later stages of the survey*

    The profiles of several key variables were compared for the second and third stages of the survey against the first stage, and the results were shown to be very similar. A slight bias by initial feeding method was noted at each stage (see Tables I.7 and I.8), and the data were subsequently weighted to correct for this.

The weighted sample

As in 1995, when results for each country are shown separately, they are weighted only to compensate for differential non-response and the over-sampling of lower social class groups. When results are based on the United Kingdom as a whole, then the additional weighting for to compensate for over-sampling in Scotland and Northern Ireland is also applied.

Table I.6
First stage response rates by social class of husband/partner at registration and by country

	England & Wales	Scotland	Northern Ireland
		Response rate (%)	
I	85	85	82
II	82	82	80
IIIN	77	83	77
IIIM	76	71	71
IV	71	75	67
V	66	69	58
Other/unclassified/no husband/partner recorded	65	58	50
All mothers	**74**	**73**	**68**

Table I.7
Response to Stage 2 by initial method feeding and country

	England & Wales	Scotland	Northern Ireland
		Response rate (%)	
Breastfed	88	87	93
Not breastfed	84	84	89
All mothers	**87**	**86**	**91**

Table I.8
Response to Stage 3 by initial method feeding and country

	England & Wales	Scotland	Northern Ireland
		Response rate (%)	
Breastfed	89	90	91
Not breastfed	83	84	87
All mothers	**87**	**88**	**89**

[1] Registration Division of ONS for England and Wales and the General Register Offices in Scotland and Northern Ireland

[2] Nathan Keyfitz. Sampling with probabilities proportional to size: adjustment for changes in probabilities. Journal of the American Statistical Association 46 (1951) p105-109. This techniques was applied as strictly as possible, however it should be noted that there has been significant re-organisation of birth districts between 1995

[3] Excluding still births and additional births resulting from multiple births

Appendix II

Composition of the 2000 sample

II.1 Comparison of the sample with population figures

Tables II.1 to II.3 show the composition of the weighted sample at Stage 1 for sex of baby, age of mothers and social class as compared with population data where this data has been available. The population figures refer to all live births registered in 2000.

On the whole, the figures show that the sample data is very similar in profile to the population data for these three attributes. Table II.1 shows that the sex of babies is similar for both sample and population, although the sample in England and Wales tended to slightly over-represent boys compared with the population (53% compared to 51%).

Table II.1
Distribution of the population and the sample by sex of the baby and country (2000)

	England & Wales		Scotland		Northern Ireland	
	Population %	Survey %	Population %	Survey %	Population %	Survey %
Male	51	53	51	50	52	51
Female	49	47	49	50	48	48
Base:	604,441	5441	53,076	2274	21,512	1778

Within all countries, the distribution of the sample for age of mother is very similar to that found in the population of all births for these countries. The age profile of the sample in England and Wales is virtually identical to the population of all births, although in Scotland and Northern Ireland there is a very slight over-representation of mothers aged 30 or over compared with the population (49% compared with 47% in Scotland, and 49% compared with 46% in Northern Ireland).

Table II.2
Distribution of the population and the sample by age of mother and country (2000)

	England & Wales		Scotland		Northern Ireland	
	Population %	Survey %	Population %	Survey %	Population %	Survey %
Under 20	8	7	9	6	8	6
20-24	18	18	17	16	17	15
25-29	28	28	28	29	29	30
30-34	30	30	31	31	30	33
35 or over	17	16	16	18	16	16
All aged 30+	46	46	47	49	46	49
Base:	604,441	5441	53,076	2274	21,512	1778

The population figures for social class are not based on all live births in 2000, but instead on the social class details of all births in the sampled period. The sample data (which is based on questionnaire responses) classifies a greater proportion of mothers to no partner or partner unclassified (19% in the UK compared with 13% of all births in the sample period which is based on social class recorded from registration records). However, once this difference is taken into account, the social class profiles of population and sample are very similar

Table II.3
Distribution of the population and the sample by social class as defined by current or last occupation of husband or partner

	England & Wales		Scotland		Northern Ireland		United Kingdom	
	Population* %	Survey %	Population %	Survey %	Population %	Survey %	Population %	Survey %
I & II	34	32	31	31	27	26	34	32
IIINM	9	9	9	9	11	10	10	9
All non-manual	**43**	**41**	**40**	**41**	**38**	**36**	**44**	**40**
IIIM	25	26	28	26	31	29	26	26
IV & V	18	15	22	16	18	14	18	15
All manual	**43**	**40**	**50**	**42**	**49**	**43**	**44**	**41**
No partner/ unclassified	13	19	10	18	13	21	13	19
Base	64250	5441	5121	2274	3947	1779	73318	9492

* In England & Wales, only 10% of births are coded to social class so the "population" data is in fact based on a 10% sample

II.2   Details of the 2000 sample

The main changes in sample composition between 1995 and 2000 are highlighted in Chapter 1. These were:

- An increase in the proportion of mothers aged 30 or over;
- An increase in the proportion of mothers educated to higher education level (aged 19+);

These changes are a continuation of trends evident since 1990. Tables II.4 to II.11 give further details of the composition of the 2000 sample compared with previous surveys (1990 and 1995).

The age of mothers both nationally and in the sample, has increased since 1995. Table II.4 shows that this increase was evident for both mothers of first and later births.

Table II.4

Distribution of the sample by mother's age, for first and later births (1990,1995 Great Britain, 2000 United Kingdom)*

	First births			Later births			All babies**		
	1990 %	1995 %	2000 %	1990 %	1995 %	2000 %	1990 %	1995 %	2000 %
Under 20	13	12	13	2	1	1	7	6	7
20-24	31	26	23	20	14	13	25	19	18
25-29	36	34	30	39	34	27	37	34	29
30-34†		22	24		34	36		28	31
35 or over†		6	9		17	22		12	16
All aged 30 or over	20	28	33	39	50	49	31	40	47
Base:	*2430*	*2271*	*4448*	*2983*	*2745*	*5044*	*5413*	*5017*	*9492*

* Note that 1990 and 1995 data based on GB and 2000 based on UK
** Includes some cases for whom exact birth order not known
† Not identified separately in 1990* Not applicable in 1995 and 2000, as there was no interviewer-administered fieldwork at Stage 1

Table II.5 shows the relationship between social class and mother's age for mothers of first babies only. There is a consistent pattern of older mothers in non-manual social class groups. Thus, in 2000, 53% of mothers in social classes I and II were aged 30 or over compared with 24% of mothers in classes IV and V. The increase in age of mothers between 1995 and 2000 was found in every social class group except IIIM. However, this increase was concentrated to a greater extent among mothers in higher social classes. For example, between 1995 and 2000 the proportion of mothers aged 30 or over in social classes I and II rose from 44% to 53%, although within social classes IV and V, the increase was only from 21% to 24%.

Appendix III
Sampling errors

III.1 Sources of error in surveys

As with any survey, estimates resulting from the Infant Feeding Study will be subject to sources or error. Sample survey theory describes two sources of error: *systematic error* (or bias) and *random error*.

Systematic error or bias arises when respondents to the survey are not representative of the universe of interest. This can arise if either the original sample selected was unrepresentative or the response rate to the survey is low and varies significantly across different groups of participants. A rigorous sample design, with a sample selected from an exhaustive sampling frame will eradicate the former, whilst a high response rate across all respondent groups will resolve difficulties of the latter type.

The Infant Feeding Survey 2000 conducted fieldwork in mainly August and September of 2000 as in previous quinquennial rounds of the study. In some cases all mothers giving birth in this period were part of the study, but the mothers in the survey are considered to a random sample of mothers to represent all mothers in 2000.

Overall, though, the main source of error is sampling error. The extent of this depends on the natural variation in any measure that is collected and the sample size achieved.

III.2 Standard errors and confidence limits

For any percentage estimate p, the 95% confidence interval for the universe statistic **P** is:

$$p +/- 1.96*se(p), \quad \text{where se(p) is the standard error of the estimate.} \tag{A}$$

The standard error of p is unknown but is estimated by the quantity:

$$\sqrt{p(1-p)/n}. \quad \text{where n is the sample size for a particular group.} \tag{B}$$

This theory applies to a total sample and for the sub-groups when the design is random, unclustered, and proportionately stratified. This is the case for the Northern Irish and Scottish surveys. However, In England and Wales the design has been clustered around certain birth registration subdistricts and at a UK level it is skewed towards Scotland and Northern Ireland. The effect of the clustering and skew means that the actual sample sizes cannot be used as 'n' in (B) and that effective sample sizes will need to be calculated and used instead.

The effective sample size is the actual sample size divided by the design effect. A design effect of one arises when a sample is completely unclustered and representative of the universe it represents. Then the effective sample size is the same as the actual sample size. This will not be the case in this survey for estimates in England and Wales because of the reasons given above. However, in Scotland in Northern Ireland the design is closer to a simple random sample and so design effects are close to one. A design effect factor (design factor = √ design effect) been derived from estimated design effects for use when calculating confidence intervals.

The design standard errors and design factors for selected Infant feeding Survey measures are given in the following tables together with weighted bases, for selected measures, in each of England & Wales, Scotland, Northern Ireland and the UK are given in Tables III (i) – III (iii). The design standard errors are usually greater than the standard errors obtained under simple random sampling and should be used when estimating confidence intervals for estimates. The design factor is the ratio of the standard error of the design to the standard error of a simple random sample of the same size. The weighted bases are given as an indication of the sample sizes in particular sub-groups but may differ from the achieved number of interviews in each sub-group, on which the calculations of design standard error and design factor are based.

For survey estimates that are not included in tables III (i) – III (iii), the 95% confidence intervals for a percentage p can be calculated using the formula:

p +/- 1.96*deft*se (p),   (C)

where se(p) is the standard error from (B) assuming a simple random sample, and the 'deft' is the design factor. A suitable value for deft can be estimated from tables III (i) – (iii), by selecting a measure in the table which is likely to be clustered in the same way and based on a similar sample size.

Design factors in Scotland and Northern Ireland will tend to be smaller than those in England & Wales because of the different designs in the countries. At a UK level design factors are a combination of all the participatory countries and will be higher than those in Scotland and Northern Ireland, but lower than those in England & Wales. Furthermore, design factors will tend to be lower for subgroups than for the sample as a whole.

As an illustration the following explains the relationship between the incidence of breastfeeding figure quoted in table III.1

Estimate, p = 70.5%.

Design standard error, dse(p) = 1.31.

Design factor, deft = 2.11

Weighted Base = 5,440

Confidence Interval = 70.5% +/-1.96*1.31 or 67.9% - 73.1%

Table III.1

Design standard errors for incidence & duration of breastfeeding: England & Wales

Characteristic	Sample sub-group	Percentage	Standard error	Design factor	Weighted base
Incidence of breastfeeding					
	Overall	70.5	1.31	2.11	5440
Birth order	First birth	75.5	1.39	1.62	2560
	Later birth	66.2	1.43	1.62	2880
Mother's age	Under 20	50.6	2.41	0.90	393
(for first babies only)	20-24	65.7	2.08	1.07	610
	25-29	80.0	1.66	1.16	751
	30 and over	88.8	1.35	1.24	823
Age mother finished	16 or under	54.7	1.31	1.77	2009
full-time education	17 or 18	72.2	1.51	1.46	1874
	19 or over	89.5	0.87	1.09	1507
Social class of husband or partner	I	91.3	1.40	0.95	369
	II	83.6	1.32	1.31	1372
	III non-manual	79.1	1.82	0.97	465
	III manual	65.3	1.56	1.22	1398
	IV	62.2	2.27	1.12	578
	V	58.5	2.88	0.36	218
	No partner	53.3	2.18	1.23	168
	Unclassified	70.7	4.05	1.15	871
Percentage of women who continued to breastfeed for at least 6 weeks after the birth					
	Overall	63.9	1.14	1.26	2898
Birth order	First birth	59.3	1.46	1.11	1440
	Later birth	68.4	1.31	1.06	1457
Mother's age (for first babies only)	Under 20	39.3	4.49	0.90	97
	20-24	45.3	2.74	0.88	263
	25-29	60.0	2.13	0.94	421
	30 and over	67.9	1.86	0.97	605
Age mother finished full-time	16 or under	51.1	1.73	0.98	810
education	17 or 18	60.1	1.36	0.89	1043
	19 or over	77.7	1.42	1.08	1022
Social class of husband or partner	I	76.2	2.57	1.00	281
	II	73.0	1.32	0.88	904
	III non-manual	66.2	2.57	0.93	298
	III manual	56.2	1.97	1.03	692
	IV	56.5	2.66	0.89	279
	V	41.4	4.16	0.78	86
	No partner	53.8	2.47	0.82	283
	Unclassified	59.9	6.02	1.04	74
Percentage of women who continued to breastfeed for at least 4 months after the birth					
	Overall	43.0	1.14	1.22	2898
Birth order	First birth	38.5	1.38	1.06	1440
	Later birth	47.4	1.40	1.06	1457
Mother's age (for first babies only)	Under 20	19.3	3.54	0.88	97
	20-24	21.9	2.14	0.84	263
	25-29	38.3	2.48	1.10	471
	30 and over	49.2	1.94	0.95	605
Age mother finished full-time	16 or under	30.0	1.70	1.07	810
education	17 or 18	37.9	1.43	0.94	1043
	19 or over	58.7	1.53	0.98	1022
Social class of husband or partner	I	61.8	3.00	1.03	281
	II	52.4	1.56	0.93	904
	III non-manual	45.7	2.48	0.85	298
	III manual	33.8	1.59	0.88	692
	IV	31.2	2.87	1.02	279
	V	31.1	3.92	0.78	86
	No partner	31.6	2.37	0.85	283
	Unclassified	35.2	5.34	0.95	74

Table III.2

Design standard errors for selected measures of sample: England & Wales

Characteristic	Sample sub-group	Percentage	Standard error	Design factor	Weighted base
During pregnancy					
Took supplementary iron or vitamins		53.9	0.91	1.34	5399
Attended antenatal classes		36.0	1.03	1.57	5404
Non-smokers					
Never smoked		51.9	0.76	1.09	5224
Gave up smoking over a year before pregnancy		12.8	0.51	1.10	5224
All smokers		35.3	0.73	1.11	5224
Smoked before pregnancy					
Gave up smoking less than a year before pregnancy		3.4	0.25	0.98	5224
Gave up smoking on confirmation of pregnancy		11.0	0.36	0.83	5224
Gave up smoking later in pregnancy, stayed quit		1.5	0.13	0.78	5224
Smoked throughout pregnancy		19.4	0.70	1.27	5224
Gave up, but started again		3.7	0.21	0.80	5224
Cut down		14.2	0.59	1.22	5224
Did not cut down		1.6	0.17	0.96	5224
Drank before pregnancy					
All stage 1 mothers		87.2	0.95	2.09	5440
Mothers age	Under 20	87.6	1.78	1.06	383
	20 - 24	83.9	1.72	1.46	973
	25 - 30	87.1	1.10	1.29	1544
	30 - 34	88.0	0.98	1.22	1647
	35 or over	90.5	1.06	1.06	873
Drank during pregnancy					
All stage 1 mothers		61.5	0.93	1.40	5440
Mothers age	Under 20	53.3	2.24	0.87	383
	20 - 24	54.2	2.02	1.26	973
	25 - 30	59.0	1.26	1.00	1544
	30 - 34	64.8	1.18	1.00	1647
	35 or over	72.3	1.50	0.98	873
Gave up drinking during pregnancy					
All stage 1 mothers		29.0	0.71	1.08	4744
Mothers age	Under 20	38.1	2.15	0.81	336
	20 - 24	34.9	1.67	1.00	816
	25 - 30	31.6	1.16	0.91	1343
	30 - 34	26.1	1.10	0.95	1449
	35 or over	19.9	1.26	0.88	789
Percentage of women who planned to breastfeed					
All mothers		92.1	0.36	0.99	5440
Birth order (mothers in UK)	First birth	91.2	0.55	0.97	2560
	Later birth	93.0	0.41	0.85	2880
Percentage of women who had given solid food to the baby by three months of age					
All mothers		22.9	0.98	1.50	4112
Method of feeding	First birth	22.8	1.12	1.17	1914
	Later birth	22.9	1.16	1.29	2198
Percentage of women who had given solid food to the baby by four months of age					
All mothers		84.9	0.60	1.07	4112
Method of feeding	First birth	87.4	0.80	1.06	1914
	Later birth	82.8	0.73	0.91	2198
Percentage of women who had given meat to baby at stage 3					
All mothers		94.1	0.39	1.06	4014

Table III.3
Design standard errors for incidence & duration of breastfeeding: Scotland

Characteristic	Sample sub-group	Percentage	Standard error	Design factor	Weighted base
Incidence of breastfeeding					
	Overall	63.0	1.03	1.02	2274
Birth order	First birth	67.0	1.42	1.01	1115
	Later birth	59.1	1.47	1.02	1159
Mother's age (for first babies only)	Under 20	31.4	3.97	0.97	148
	20-24	55.2	3.25	1.01	247
	25-29	70.8	2.44	1.04	358
	30 and over	82.6	2.01	1.03	368
Age mother finished full-time education	16 or under	45.6	1.77	1.01	813
	17 or 18	63.0	1.82	1.03	743
	19 or over	83.5	1.42	1.02	708
Social class of husband or partner	I	89.9	2.40	1.01	162
	II	79.2	1.76	1.02	553
	III non-manual	65.2	3.37	1.01	206
	III manual	57.4	2.18	1.08	598
	IV	58.2	3.31	1.06	247
	V	47.0	4.02	0.85	112
	No partner	65.0	2.57	0.97	393
	Unclassified	40.7	5.56	0.86	54
Percentage of women who continued to breastfeed for at least 6 weeks after the birth					
	Overall	66.2	1.46	1.01	1093
Birth order	First birth	61.0	2.13	1.01	550
	Later birth	71.4	1.98	1.01	544
Mother's age (for first babies only)	Under 20	46.6	11.74	0.96	17
	20-24	40.2	5.98	1.01	69
	25-29	62.8	3.47	1.02	207
	30 and over	66.0	3.04	1.01	255
Age mother finished full-time education	16 or under	56.0	3.11	1.02	263
	17 or 18	59.1	2.69	1.02	353
	19 or over	77.0	1.98	0.99	475
Social class of husband or partner	I	82.7	3.44	0.99	120
	II	70.7	2.47	1.01	354
	III non-manual	69.5	4.39	1.00	112
	III manual	59.9	3.29	1.07	260
	IV	66.5	4.98	1.04	99
	V	47.3	6.85	0.85	39
	No partner	44.0	5.19	0.97	87
	Unclassified	81.7	7.51	0.90	22
Percentage of women who continued to breastfeed for at least 4 months after the birth					
	Overall	49.0	1.55	1.01	1093
Birth order	First birth	43.1	2.17	1.02	550
	Later birth	54.9	2.18	1.01	544
Mother's age (for first babies only)	Under 20	27.8	10.70	0.98	17
	20-24	23.7	5.17	1.00	69
	25-29	41.7	3.53	1.02	207
	30 and over	50.3	3.21	1.01	255
Age mother finished full-time education	16 or under	35.9	3.02	1.01	263
	17 or 18	39.7	2.67	1.02	353
	19 or over	63.2	2.26	1.01	475
Social class of husband or partner	I	65.6	4.35	0.99	120
	II	54.3	2.70	1.01	354
	III non-manual	54.4	4.75	1.00	112
	III manual	42.3	3.31	1.07	260
	IV	41.8	5.22	1.04	99
	V	34.7	6.62	0.86	39
	No partner	29.9	4.82	0.97	87
	Unclassified	55.7	9.21	0.86	22

Table III.4

Design standard errors for selected measures of sample: Scotland

Characteristic	Sample sub-group	Percentage	Standard error	Design factor	Weighted base
During pregnancy					
Took supplementary iron or vitamins		52.4	1.07	1.02	2261
Attended antenatal classes		46.5	1.07	1.02	2260
Non-smokers					
Never smoked		52.4	1.08	1.02	2206
Gave up smoking over a year before pregnancy		11.2	0.68	1.02	2206
All smokers		36.4	1.04	1.01	2206
Smoked before pregnancy					
Gave up smoking less than a year before pregnancy		3.0	0.37	1.02	2206
Gave up smoking on confirmation of pregnancy		9.3	0.63	1.01	2206
Gave up smoking later in pregnancy, stayed quit		2.0	0.30	1.02	2206
Smoked throughout pregnancy		22.1	0.89	1.01	2206
Gave up, but started again		4.8	0.46	1.00	2206
Cut down		15.0	0.76	1.00	2206
Did not cut down		2.3	0.33	1.02	2206
Drank before pregnancy					
All stage 1 mothers		89.3	0.66	1.01	2274
Mothers age	Under 20	82.9	3.03	0.96	143
	20 - 24	88.5	1.69	1.01	360
	25 - 30	90.4	1.16	1.01	655
	30 - 34	90.1	1.15	1.03	710
	35 or over	89.3	1.57	1.02	402
Drank during pregnancy					
All stage 1 mothers		58.7	1.06	1.02	2274
Mothers age	Under 20	40.9	3.98	0.96	143
	20 - 24	56.5	2.65	1.00	360
	25 - 30	54.4	2.01	1.03	655
	30 - 34	63.9	1.86	1.03	710
	35 or over	65.2	2.43	1.02	402
Gave up drinking during pregnancy					
All stage 1 mothers		33.8	1.07	1.02	2031
Mothers age	Under 20	49.4	4.43	0.96	119
	20 - 24	35.4	2.69	1.00	319
	25 - 30	39.5	2.07	1.03	592
	30 - 34	29.0	1.85	1.03	640
	35 or over	26.5	2.36	1.01	359
Percentage of women who planned to breastfeed					
All mothers		90.5	0.63	1.02	2274
Birth order (mothers in UK)	First birth	88.1	0.98	1.01	1115
	Later birth	92.8	0.8	1.02	1159
Percentage of women who had given solid food to the baby by three months of age					
All mothers		27.6	1.1	1.02	1718
Method of feeding	First birth	29.0	1.61	1.02	824
	Later birth	26.3	1.50	1.02	894
Percentage of women who had given solid food to the baby by four months of age					
All mothers		83.5	0.91	1.01	1718
Method of feeding	First birth	85.1	1.25	1.01	824
	Later birth	81.9	1.30	1.01	894
Percentage of women who had given meat to baby at stage 3					
All mothers		91.5	0.69	1.02	1696

Table III.5
Design standard errors for incidence & duration of breastfeeding: Northern Ireland

Characteristic	Sample sub-group	Percentage	Standard error	Design factor	Weighted base
Incidence of breastfeeding					
	Overall	54.2	1.19	1.01	1778
Birth order	First birth	59.1	1.83	1.00	729
	Later birth	50.8	1.55	1.01	1049
Mother's age (for first babies only)	Under 20	25.9	4.47	0.99	99
	20-24	42.2	3.70	1.00	180
	25-29	68.9	3.14	1.02	220
	30 and over	76.0	2.85	1.02	231
Age mother finished full-time education	16 or under	37.9	2.31	1.01	446
	17 or 18	50.3	1.88	1.01	716
	19 or over	71.1	1.85	1.00	603
Social class of husband or partner	I	86.3	3.41	0.97	96
	II	68.4	2.39	0.99	369
	III non-manual	66.1	3.54	1.00	179
	III manual	52.0	2.27	1.03	519
	IV	50.4	3.83	1.04	186
	V	37.7	6.08	0.93	55
	No partner	46.0	2.48	0.99	349
	Unclassified	32.5	9.44	0.95	25
Percentage of women who continued to breastfeed for at least 6 weeks after the birth					
	Overall	49.2	1.79	1.00	787
Birth order	First birth	43.6	2.65	1.00	352
	Later birth	53.8	2.40	1.00	435
Mother's age (for first babies only)	Under 20	18.3	9.65	0.98	17
	20-24	30.2	5.99	0.99	69
	25-29	42.8	4.37	1.01	207
	30 and over	52.2	4.14	1.00	255
Age mother finished full-time education	16 or under	40.0	4.45	1.01	124
	17 or 18	43.6	2.93	1.01	293
	19 or over	56.8	2.58	1.00	367
Social class of husband or partner	I	75.9	4.83	0.97	73
	II	54.7	3.35	0.98	214
	III non-manual	42.0	5.12	1.00	92
	III manual	46.1	3.47	1.03	221
	IV	45.7	5.90	1.04	78
	V	43.6	11.79	0.92	15
	No partner	31.5	5.10	1.00	83
	Unclassified	54.4	15.05	0.94	10
Percentage of women who continued to breastfeed for at least 4 months after the birth					
	Overall	27.4	1.60	1.00	787
Birth order	First birth	21.7	2.21	1.00	352
	Later birth	32.0	2.24	1.00	435
Mother's age (for first babies only)	Under 20	7.1	6.79	1.04	15
	20-24	15.2	4.71	1.00	58
	25-29	23.1	3.71	1.01	132
	30 and over	24.5	3.56	1.00	147
Age mother finished full-time education	16 or under	22.1	3.77	1.01	124
	17 or 18	21.4	2.42	1.01	293
	19 or over	34.0	2.47	1.00	367
Social class of husband or partner	I	45.2	5.64	0.97	73
	II	32.3	3.14	0.98	214
	III non-manual	20.5	4.20	1.00	92
	III manual	24.2	2.98	1.03	221
	IV	25.1	5.13	1.04	78
	V	10.3	6.96	0.89	15
	No partner	17.2	4.20	1.01	83
	Unclassified	54.4	15.05	0.94	10

Table III.6

Design standard errors for selected measures of sample: Northern Ireland

Characteristic	Sample sub-group	Percentage	Standard error	Design factor	Weighted base
During pregnancy					
Took supplementary iron or vitamins		71.6	1.08	1.01	1770
Attended antenatal classes		32.0	1.11	1.01	1771
Non-smokers					
Never smoked		53.7	1.21	1.00	1722
Gave up smoking over a year before pregnancy		10.0	0.73	1.01	1722
All smokers		36.3	1.16	1.00	1722
Smoked before pregnancy					
Gave up smoking less than a year before pregnancy		2.9	0.41	1.00	1722
Gave up smoking on confirmation of pregnancy		10.0	0.73	1.01	1722
Gave up smoking later in pregnancy, stayed quit		0.8	0.21	1.02	1722
Smoked throughout pregnancy		22.5	1.01	1.00	1722
Gave up, but started again		4.2	0.48	1.00	1722
Cut down		15.5	0.87	1.00	1722
Did not cut down		2.8	0.40	1.00	1722
Drank before pregnancy					
All stage 1 mothers		82.4	0.91	1.01	1778
Mothers age	Under 20	84.2	3.54	0.99	103
	20 - 24	87.8	1.98	0.99	269
	25 - 30	83.9	1.62	1.01	526
	30 - 34	79.7	1.67	1.01	589
	35 or over	80.3	2.37	1.01	284
Drank during pregnancy					
All stage 1 mothers		51.8	1.20	1.00	1778
Mothers age	Under 20	49.3	4.82	0.98	103
	20 - 24	41.8	3.01	0.99	269
	25 - 30	51.5	2.21	1.01	526
	30 - 34	53.3	2.09	1.01	589
	35 or over	60.3	2.92	1.00	284
Gave up drinking during pregnancy					
All stage 1 mothers		36.6	1.27	1.01	1464
Mothers age	Under 20	41.5	5.17	0.98	87
	20 - 24	51.5	3.24	1.00	236
	25 - 30	38.3	2.34	1.01	441
	30 - 34	32.6	2.19	1.01	469
	35 or over	24.6	2.85	1.00	228
Percentage of women who planned to breastfeed					
All mothers		90.8	0.7	1.00	1778
Birth order (mothers in UK)	First birth	85.7	1.3	1.00	729
	Later birth	94.4	0.7	1.00	1049
Percentage of women who had given solid food to the baby by three months of age					
All mothers		34.4	1.26	1.01	1437
Method of feeding	First birth	35.5	1.98	1.00	984
	Later birth	33.6	1.63	1.01	852
Percentage of women who had given solid food to the baby by four months of age					
All mothers		84.5	1.0	1.01	1437
Method of feeding	First birth	87.2	1.39	1.00	584
	Later birth	82.7	1.31	1.01	852
Percentage of women who had given meat to baby at stage 3					
All mothers		90.1	0.81	1.02	1405

Table III.7

Design standard errors for incidence & duration of breastfeeding: United Kingdom

Characteristic	Sample sub-group	Percentage	Standard error	Design factor	Weighted base
Incidence of breastfeeding					
	Overall	69.1	0.68	1.20	9492
Birth order	First birth	74.1	1.43	1.48	4448
	Later birth	64.7	1.45	1.47	5044
Mother's age (for first babies only)	Under 20	48.2	2.34	1.09	594
	20-24	63.8	2.23	1.22	1025
	25-29	78.8	1.86	1.29	1353
	30 and over	87.7	1.55	1.33	1461
Age mother finished full-time education	16 or under	53.5	1.46	1.29	3436
	17 or 18	70.2	1.59	1.41	3289
	19 or over	87.8	0.94	1.24	2683
Social class of husband or partner	I	91.0	1.48	1.14	639
	II	82.6	1.47	1.36	2366
	III non-manual	77.3	1.92	1.16	823
	III manual	64.0	1.77	1.34	2461
	IV	61.3	2.51	1.28	1010
	V	56.9	2.61	1.02	382
	No partner	69.7	2.00	1.31	279
	Unclassified	51.1	4.72	1.22	1532
Percentage of women who continued to breastfeed for at least 6 weeks after the birth					
	Overall	63.4	1.30	1.36	4976
Birth order	First birth	58.7	1.62	1.26	2464
	Later birth	67.9	1.42	1.22	2512
Mother's age (for first babies only)	Under 20	38.8	4.94	1.08	158
	20-24	45.7	2.94	1.08	439
	25-29	59.2	2.25	1.14	818
	30 and over	70.9	1.93	1.16	1041
Age mother finished full-time education	16 or under	51.1	1.95	1.16	1350
	17 or 18	59.3	1.44	1.09	1783
	19 or over	76.4	1.40	1.23	1806
Social class of husband or partner	I	76.7	2.65	1.16	486
	II	72.2	1.39	1.09	1546
	III non-manual	65.1	2.70	1.12	516
	III manual	55.9	2.18	1.22	1198
	IV	56.6	2.84	1.10	478
	V	41.9	3.76	0.95	148
	No partner	52.2	2.49	1.03	482
	Unclassified	60.9	6.49	1.17	122
Percentage of women who continued to breastfeed for at least 4 months after the birth					
	Overall	42.7	1.29	1.34	4976
Birth order	First birth	38.2	1.51	1.22	2464
	Later birth	47.1	1.51	1.22	2512
Mother's age (for first babies only)	Under 20	18.8	3.87	1.07	164
	20-24	25.1	2.35	1.03	657
	25-29	38.2	2.64	1.23	1366
	30 and over	50.6	2.06	1.16	2767
Age mother finished full-time education	16 or under	30.2	1.97	1.21	1350
	17 or 18	37.3	1.59	1.14	1783
	19 or over	57.6	1.57	1.17	1806
Social class of husband or partner	I	61.3	3.15	1.18	486
	II	51.7	1.65	1.12	1546
	III non-manual	44.9	2.52	1.06	516
	III manual	33.8	1.69	1.10	1198
	IV	31.5	3.21	1.21	478
	V	30.8	3.53	0.95	148
	No partner	30.8	2.41	1.05	482
	Unclassified	36.7	5.54	1.09	122

Table III.8

Design standard errors for selected measures of sample: United Kingdom

Characteristic	Sample sub-group	Percentage	Standard error	Design factor	Weighted base
During pregnancy					
Took supplementary iron or vitamins		54.7	0.96	1.37	9424
Attended antenatal classes		36.5	1.06	1.96	9431
Non-smokers					
Never smoked		52.1	0.79	1.24	9126
Gave up smoking over a year before pregnancy		12.5	0.53	1.25	9126
All smokers		35.4	0.77	1.25	9126
Smoked before pregnancy					
Gave up smoking less than a year before pregnancy		3.3	0.25	1.17	9126
Gave up smoking on confirmation of pregnancy		10.8	0.35	1.05	9126
Gave up smoking later in pregnancy, stayed quit		1.5	0.13	1.07	9126
Smoked throughout pregnancy		19.8	0.72	1.32	9126
Gave up, but started again		3.8	0.21	1.02	9126
Cut down		14.3	0.61	1.31	9126
Did not cut down		1.7	0.18	1.55	9126
Drank before pregnancy					
All stage 1 mothers		87.1	0.86	1.88	9492
Mothers age	Under 20	87.2	0.38	1.06	8394
	20 - 24	84.3	0.79	1.46	1670
	25 - 30	87.1	0.57	1.29	2703
	30 - 34	87.6	0.50	1.22	2894
	35 or over	89.8	0.35	1.06	1534
Drank during pregnancy					
All stage 1 mothers		60.7	0.98	1.39	9492
Mothers age	Under 20	52.3	0.94	1.35	657
	20 - 24	53.7	1.97	1.95	1670
	25 - 30	58.1	1.22	1.55	2703
	30 - 34	64.0	1.20	1.55	2894
	35 or over	71.1	1.09	1.53	1534
Gave up drinking during pregnancy					
All stage 1 mothers		29.8	0.77	1.23	8266
Mothers age	Under 20	39.0	0.56	1.02	573
	20 - 24	35.7	0.73	1.17	1408
	25 - 30	32.6	0.65	1.12	2353
	30 - 34	26.7	0.64	1.15	2536
	35 or over	20.6	0.53	1.09	1377
Percentage of women who planned to breastfeed					
All mothers		91.8	0.39	1.17	9492
Birth order (mothers in UK)	First birth	90.6	0.40	1.16	4448
	Later birth	92.9	0.30	1.07	5044
Percentage of women who had given solid food to the baby by three months of age					
All mothers		23.8	1.02	1.43	7267
Method of feeding	First birth	23.9	0.82	1.28	796
	Later birth	23.8	0.91	1.35	3900
Percentage of women who had given solid food to the baby by four months of age					
All mothers		84.8	0.63	1.23	7267
Method of feeding	First birth	87.2	0.58	1.22	796
	Later birth	82.7	0.55	1.11	9900
Percentage of women who had given meat to baby at stage 3					
All mothers		93.7	0.43	1.22	7100

Appendix IV

Registration subdistricts sampled in England & Wales

No	District	Subdistrict	Subdistrict name	No	District	Subdistrict	Subdistrict name
1.	7	1	Oldham	53.	465	1	Braintree
2.	9	1	Rochdale	54.	466	1	Basildon
3.	11	1	Salford	55.	468	1	Chelmsford
4.	14	1	Tameside	56.	479	1	Cheltenham
5.	15	1	Trafford	57.	491	1	Basingstoke
6.	18	1	Wigan & Leigh	58.	497	1	Portsmouth
7.	23	1	Knowsley	59.	501	2	Gosport
8.	25	1	Liverpool	60.	517	1	Kidderminster
9.	45	1	Rotherham	61.	527	1	Worcester
10.	48	1	Sheffield	62.	532	1	Hatfield
11.	51	1	Gateshead	63.	536	1	Watford
12.	54	1	North Tyneside	64.	542	1	Beverley
13.	63	1	Coventry	65.	544	1	Bridlington
14.	70	1	Sandwell	66.	548	1	NE Lincolnshire
15.	73	1	Solihull South	67.	550	1	Hull
16.	77	1	Wolverhampton	68.	556	1	Isle Of Wight
17.	82	1	Keighley	69.	560	1	Canterbury with Swale
18.	89	1	Huddersfield	70.	562	1	Thames
19.	92	1	Leeds	71.	575	1	Thanet with Dover
20.	99	1	Wakefield	72.	581	1	Blackpool
21.	218	1	Barking&Dagenham	73.	583	1	Chorley
22.	229	1	Greenwich	74.	586	2	Rossendale
23.	231	1	Hammersmith	75.	587	2	Lancaster
24.	238	1	Islington	76.	610	1	Boston
25.	240	1	Kingston-U-Thames	77.	616	1	Grantham
26.	241	1	Lambeth	78.	636	1	Great Yarmouth
27.	247	1	Redbridge	79.	685*	1	Beeston & Stapleford
28.	250	1	Camden	80.	685*	2	Carlton
29.	251	1	Southwark	81.	685*	3	Eastwood
30.	255	1	Waltham Forest	82.	689	1	Nottingham
31.	257	1	Newham	83.	691	1	Worksop
32.	300	1	Bath	84.	702	1	Oxford
33.	301	1	Bristol	85.	710*	1	Bridgnorth
34.	322	1	Ascot	86.	715	1	Shrewsbury
35.	322	3	Windsor	87.	721	1	Frome
36.	326	1	Milton Keynes	88.	724	1	Taunton
37.	327	1	Chiltern Hills	89.	732	1	Lichfield
38.	333	1	Huntingdon	90.	735	1	Stafford
39.	340	1	Cheshire West	91.	737	1	Stoke-On-Trent
40.	348	1	Middlesbrough	92.	757	1	North Surrey
41.	350	1	Stockton-on-Tees	93.	761	1	West Surrey
42.	351	1	Hartlepool	94.	768	1	Nuneaton& Bedworth
43.	370	1	Truro	95.	770	1	Rugby
44.	377	1	Kendal	96.	780	1	Crawley
45.	391*	2	Matlock	97.	781	1	Haywards Heath
46.	393	1	Chesterfield	98.	788	1	Chippenham
47.	416	1	Plymouth	99.	795	1	Salisbury
48.	421	1	Mid Devon	100.	816	1	Aberystwyth
49.	442	1	Durham Western	101.	818	1	Carmarthen
50.	454	1	Eastbourne	102.	841	1	Ogwen
51.	456	1	Hastings & Rother	103.	890	1	Cardiff/Caerdydd
52.	461	1	Uckfield	104.	896	1	Neath

* Combined into one area

Appendix V

Coding frame for types of drinks

Water

Water from the tap

Boiled tap water

Mineral water (include "with a hint ofs...")

Purified water (bought from a shop)

Other water not otherwise specified

Water with sugar/honey added

Water with sugar added

Water with honey added

Baby drink with added sugar/glucose

Baby drink with added sugar/glucose (specified)

Baby drink unsweetened

Diluted concentrate Baby juice drink

Ready to Drink Baby juice drink

Other unsweetened baby drink – not specified as ready to drink or concentrate

Other baby drinks not otherwise specified

All other baby drinks not specified above.

Commercial baby herbal drinks

Fennel

Orange & clove

Camomile

Lemon, barley & camomile

Peach & herb

Hibiscus, apple & rosehip

Other commercial baby herbal drink

Homemade herbal or other drinks

Homemade herbal drinks with sugar/honey added

Homemade herbal drinks, unsweetened

All homemade herbal drinks not otherwise specified

All other (non-herbal) homemade drinks not otherwise specified

Adult drink with sugar/glucose

Adult Ribena

Diluted concentrate Ribena (not specified as light)

Ready to Drink Ribena (not specified as light) including Ribena Spring

Ribena - not otherwise specified as light, dilute or ready to drink

Diluted concentrate Ribena Light

Ready to drink Ribena Light

Ribena Light – not specified as dilute or ready to drink

Ribena Toothkind (no added sugar) concentrate

Ribena Toothkind (no added sugar) ready to drink

Other adult drinks with added sugar/glucose

Sweetened fruit juice e.g. Britvic juices

Dilute concentrate squash drinks (not low calorie or diet)

Ready to drink squash drinks

Other adult drinks with added sugar/glucose not specified as ready to drink or concentrate

Adult drinks with artificial sweetener

Dilute concentrate squash drinks with artificial sweetener

Ready to drink squash drinks with artificial sweetener

"Diet" carbonated drinks

Other drinks with artificial sweetener not specified as ready to drink or concentrate

Adult drinks unsweetened

Fresh fruit juice

Diluted squash sugar/artificial sweetener free

Ready to drink squash sugar/artificial sweetener free

Other unsweetened drink not specified as ready to drink or concentrate

Other adult drink not otherwise specified

All other unspecified adult drinks.

Other drink

Tea with milk, no sugar

Tea with milk and sugar/honey

Tea with sugar/honey, no milk

Tea with neither milk nor sugar

Tea not otherwise specified

Fruit or herbal tea (caffeine free)

Fruit/herbal tea with no sugar/honey

Fruit/herbal tea with sugar/honey

Fruit or herbal tea not otherwise specified

Any other drink not elsewhere specified

Appendix VI

Coding frame for types of food

Table 9.9

Rice cereal

Baby rice (dried, in can/jars, other)

All adult rice products

Other cereal

Baby cereal (dried, cans/jars)

All types cooked at home 9adult)

Porridge (adult, homemade or commercially prepared)

Pasta (adult)

Pasta with cheese (adult)

Pasta with vegetables (adult)

Other cereal products not otherwise specified (adult, homemade or commercially prepared)

Rusk

Dried babyfood

Savoury dried babyfood

Dessert dried babyfood

Other dried babyfood

Babyfood in cans or jars

Savoury babyfood in cans/jars

Dessert babyfood canned/jars

Other cans/jars

Homemade food

All fresh/homemade foods

Other food

All non-baby commercial (ready to eat/heat & serve) foods

Table 9.10

Yoghurt

Yoghurt (homemade or commercially prepared)

Fresh fruit

Cooked fresh fruit

Raw fresh fruit

Other dessert

Homemade/commercially prepared rice pudding/semolina

Homemade/commercially prepared custard/egg custard

Other homemade desserts not otherwise specified

Ice cream

Instant whip/jellies

All other puddings/desserts not otherwise specified

Dried fruit or nuts

Nuts

Mixed dried fruit & nuts

Dried fruit

Fruit not otherwise specified

Egg

Whole egg

Egg yolk only

Cheese & dairy produce

Cheese

Cheese sauce

Other/mixed dairy products not otherwise specified

Meat based meal

Beef/chicken/turkey/lamb/pork/bacon (including with vegetables/rice/pasta/ pastry or pies)

Meat based stew/casserole/chilli/spaghetti bolognese

Meat based soup (homemade or commercially prepared)

Meat based gravy

Meat based ready made meals (with veg/rice/pasta/pastry/pie) including sausages & beans

Meat pizza

Other meat/mixed meal

Fish based meal

Fish based meals (including with vegetables/rice/pasta/ pastry or pies)

Fish fingers (including with veg/rice/pasta)

Fish based ready made meals (with veg/rice/pasta/pastry/pie)

Vegetable based meal

Vegetable based stew/casserole/pie/pastry

Vegetable based soup (homemade or commercially prepared)

Vegetable based gravy

Vegetable based ready made meals (with rice/pasta/pie/pastry)

Vegetable pizza

Potatoes

Potatoes (boiled, baked, fried with/without oil/butter – include oven chips etc.)

Other vegetables

All other types cooked

All other types raw

Tomato or other veg sauce

All other types of vegetable not otherwise specified

Baked beans

Other beans

Bread/toast

Slices of bread/bread & butter/margarine

Cheese sandwich

Egg sandwich

Meat sandwich

Vegetable sandwich

Yeast extract sandwich

Bread & jam/honey

Other sandwich not otherwise specified

Other foods

Other homemade food not otherwise specified

Soya protein

Ready made meals (sausages/burgers/mince)

Pizza n.e.s.

All other ready made meals n.e.s.

Homemade cakes & biscuits

Commercially prepared cakes & biscuits

Sweets

Chocolate

Crisps/savoury snacks

All other confectionery not otherwise specified

Soups n.e.s.

Commercial food products not otherwise specified

Appendix VII

Survey documents

Covering letters

There were several different versions of covering letters depending on the stage of the survey, whether it was an initial approach or a reminder, and depending on which country the mother lived in. At **Stage 1**, when the initial approach was made from the respective registration offices, there were separate versions for each of England & Wales, Scotland and Northern Ireland. Within each of these countries, there were four letters – an initial letter and three reminders. At **Stages 2 and 3** when the fieldwork in England, Wales and Scotland was handled fully by BMRB, there were three letters (initial & 2 reminders) for these countries, and an additional three letters from NISRA for the addresses in Northern Ireland.

Three letters have been appended here:

- the initial letter at Stage 1 for sampled addresses in England & Wales

- the initial letter at Stage 2 for sampled addresses in England & Wales and Scotland

- the initial letter at Stage 3 for sampled addresses in England & Wales and Scotland

Questionnaires

At Stage 1, there were three different versions of the questionnaire, one for each country. The only differences between the country versions were that the question asking about mother's ethnic background was tailored to the different countries (in line with the 2001 Census) and the NI version had an additional question about religion.

At Stages 2 and 3, there was no tailoring to country. However, there were two different versions of the questionnaire depending on whether the mother had been breastfeeding or bottle-feeding at the previous survey stage. The "bottle-feeding" versions differed from the "breastfeeding" versions only in that Q3-Q5 were omitted at Stage 2 and Q3-Q6 were omitted at Stage 3.

Three questionnaires have been appended here:

- the Stage 1 questionnaire sent to all mothers in England in Wales

- the Stage 2 questionnaire sent to all mothers who had been breastfeeding at Stage 1

- the Stage 3 questionnaire sent to all mothers who had been breastfeeding at Stage 2

Stage 1

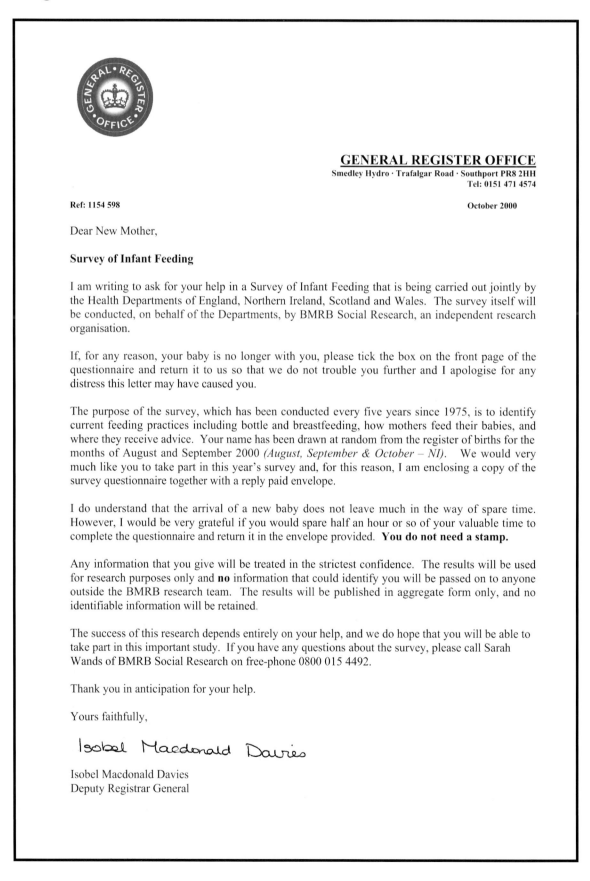

GENERAL REGISTER OFFICE
Smedley Hydro · Trafalgar Road · Southport PR8 2HH
Tel: 0151 471 4574

Ref: 1154 598

October 2000

Dear New Mother,

Survey of Infant Feeding

I am writing to ask for your help in a Survey of Infant Feeding that is being carried out jointly by the Health Departments of England, Northern Ireland, Scotland and Wales. The survey itself will be conducted, on behalf of the Departments, by BMRB Social Research, an independent research organisation.

If, for any reason, your baby is no longer with you, please tick the box on the front page of the questionnaire and return it to us so that we do not trouble you further and I apologise for any distress this letter may have caused you.

The purpose of the survey, which has been conducted every five years since 1975, is to identify current feeding practices including bottle and breastfeeding, how mothers feed their babies, and where they receive advice. Your name has been drawn at random from the register of births for the months of August and September 2000 *(August, September & October – NI)*. We would very much like you to take part in this year's survey and, for this reason, I am enclosing a copy of the survey questionnaire together with a reply paid envelope.

I do understand that the arrival of a new baby does not leave much in the way of spare time. However, I would be very grateful if you would spare half an hour or so of your valuable time to complete the questionnaire and return it in the envelope provided. **You do not need a stamp.**

Any information that you give will be treated in the strictest confidence. The results will be used for research purposes only and **no** information that could identify you will be passed on to anyone outside the BMRB research team. The results will be published in aggregate form only, and no identifiable information will be retained.

The success of this research depends entirely on your help, and we do hope that you will be able to take part in this important study. If you have any questions about the survey, please call Sarah Wands of BMRB Social Research on free-phone 0800 015 4492.

Thank you in anticipation for your help.

Yours faithfully,

Isobel Macdonald Davies

Isobel Macdonald Davies
Deputy Registrar General

Stage 2

1154598/Stage 3
Ref: SN xxxxx

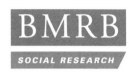

MAILMERGE NAME
MAILMERGE ADDRESS 1
ADDRESS 2
ADDRESS 3
ADDRESS 4

January 2001

Dear [NAME OF RESPONDENT],

Survey of Infant Feeding

We contacted you a few months ago asking for your help with a study of Infant Feeding which is being carried out by BMRB Social Research on behalf of the Health Departments of England, Northern Ireland, Scotland and Wales. On that occasion, you kindly completed our questionnaire and I am writing to ask if you would help us again.

The purpose of this survey is to find out how the pattern of feeding babies changes as babies get older and I am enclosing a questionnaire about this which can be returned in the reply-paid envelope provided. **You do not need a stamp.**

If, for any reason, your baby is no longer with you, please tick the box on the front page of the questionnaire and return it to us so that we do not trouble you further and I apologise for the distress this letter may have caused you.

Any information that you give will be treated in the strictest confidence. The results will be used for research purposes only and **no** information which could identify you will be passed on to anyone outside the BMRB research team. The results will be published as statistical summaries only, and no identifiable information will be retained.

The success of the survey depends on getting a reply from as many of the mothers we have written to as possible, and we do hope that you help us with the second part of this important study. If you have any questions about the survey, please call Emma Watson on free-phone 0800 015 4492.

Thank you in anticipation of your help.

Yours sincerely,

Sarah Wands
Senior Researcher Officer

BMRB International
Hadley House
79–81 Uxbridge Road
Ealing
London W5 5SU

Telephone
+44 (0)20 8566 5000

Facsimile
+44 (0)20 8579 9208

Website
www.bmrb.co.uk

BMRB International Limited
Registered in England
Number 275304
Registered office as above

Stage 3

1154598/Stage 3
Ref: SN xxxxx

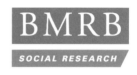

MAILMERGE NAME
MAILMERGE ADDRESS 1
ADDRESS 2
ADDRESS 3
ADDRESS 4

June 2001

Dear [NAME OF RESPONDENT],

Survey of Infant Feeding

We contacted you a few months ago asking for your help with a study of Infant Feeding that is being carried out by BMRB Social Research on behalf of the Health Departments of England, Northern Ireland, Scotland and Wales. On that occasion you kindly completed our questionnaire and now that your baby is a little older, I am writing to ask if you would help us again.

The purpose of this survey is to find out how the pattern of feeding babies changes as babies get older and the results of this survey will feed directly into Government policy. I am enclosing a questionnaire about this for you to return in the reply-paid envelope provided. **You do not need a stamp.**

If, for any reason, your baby is no longer with you, please tick the box on the front page of the questionnaire and return it to us so that we do not trouble you further and I apologise for the distress this letter may have caused you.

Any information that you give will be treated in the strictest confidence. The results will be used for research purposes only and **no** information that could identify you will be passed on to anyone outside the BMRB research team. The results will be published as statistical summaries only, and no identifiable information will be retained.

The success of the survey depends on getting a reply from as many of the mothers we have written to as possible, and we do hope that you will help us with the third and final part of this important study. If you have any questions about the survey, please call Karin Paice on free-phone 0800 015 4492.

Thank you in anticipation of your help.

Yours sincerely,

Sarah Wands
Senior Researcher Officer

BMRB International
Hadley House
79–81 Uxbridge Road
Ealing
London W5 5SU

Telephone
+44 (0)20 8566 5000

Facsimile
+44 (0)20 8579 9208

Website
www.bmrb.co.uk

EUROQUEST

KMR
Kantar Media Research

WalkerInformation
Global Network

BMRB International Limited
Registered in England
Number 275304
Registered office as above

1154-598 England/Wales

BMRB
INTERNATIONAL

Survey of Infant Feeding
October/November 2000

A

IN CONFIDENCE

What is the questionnaire about?

This questionnaire asks about you and your new baby.

If, rather than a single baby, you have twins or triplets, please answer the questionnaire in relation to the one who was born first.

If, for any reason, your baby is no longer with you, please cross the box below and return the questionnaire to us so we do not trouble you further.

My baby is no longer with me ☐

Our guarantee of confidentiality

The names and addresses of people who co-operate in surveys are held in strict confidence by BMRB. We will never pass your name or address to any Government Department, business, the media or members of the public.

How to fill in the questionnaire

1. Most questions on the following pages can be answered simply by putting a cross in the box next to the answer that applies to you.

   Example: Yes ☒
   No ☐

   Sometimes you are asked to write in a number or the answer in your own words. Please enter numbers as figures rather than words.

2. Occasionally you may have more than one answer to a question. Please cross all the boxes next to the answers that apply to you if the instruction **"Please cross one or more boxes"** is printed on top of the boxes.

   1

---

3. Sometimes you are asked to give an age or a length of time in weeks and days, or days and hours. Please follow the instructions very carefully.

   For example:

   How old is your baby?

   If your baby is 6 weeks and 2 days old enter the number of whole weeks plus any additional days

   Please enter numbers in both boxes

   6 weeks and 2 days

4. Usually after answering each question you go on to the next one unless a box you have crossed has an arrow next to it with an instruction to go to another question.

   Example: Yes ☒ ⇒ **Go to Q8**
   No ☐

   By following the arrows carefully you will miss out some questions which do not apply, so the amount you have to fill in will make the questionnaire shorter than it looks.

5. If you cannot remember, do not know, or are unable to answer a particular question please write that in.

6. When you have finished please post the questionnaire to us as soon as possible in the reply-paid envelope provided, even if you were not able to answer all of it.

   We are very grateful for your help

   2

Section 1: About your baby

First of all we would like to ask some general questions before finding out how you feed your baby at present.

Q1. What is your baby's first name?
Please write in below - 1 letter per box.

[ ][ ][ ][ ][ ][ ][ ][ ][ ][ ][ ]

Q2. How old is your baby?

Write in how many whole weeks plus any additional days   Please write numbers in both boxes

[ ] weeks   and   [ ] days

Q3. Is your baby a boy or a girl?

Boy [ ]
Girl [ ]

Q4. Is this your first baby?

Yes [ ] ⇧ **Go to Q5**
No [ ] ⇧ **Go to a)**

a). How many children do you have in total?
Please exclude stepchildren or foster children.

[ ] Write in number

3

Q5. Is your baby one of twins, triplets or other multiple birth?

No, neither [ ]
Yes, twin [ ]
Yes, triplets or other multiple birth [ ]

If you have twins or triplets please complete this questionnaire with respect to the one that was born first.

Section 2: About the milk that you give your baby

Q6. At the moment is your baby . . .

breast fed [ ]   ⇧ **Go to (a)**
bottle fed [ ]   ⇧ **Go to Q7**
or both? [ ]   ⇧ **Go to Q10**

(a). Do you ever give your baby milk in a bottle at present (apart from expressed breast milk)?

Yes (even if only occasionally) [ ]   ⇧ **Go to Q10**
No [ ]   ⇧ **Go to Q15**

Q7. Did you ever put your baby to the breast?

Yes (even if it was once only) [ ]   ⇧ **Go to Q8**
No, never [ ]   ⇧ **Go to Q10**

4

Q10. Which kind of milk do you give your baby most of the time at the moment?

*Please cross
one box only*

Cow and Gate Premium ☐

Cow and Gate Plus ☐

Cow and Gate Omneo Comfort 1 ☐

SMA Gold ☐

SMA White ☐

Milupa Milumil ☐

Milupa Aptamil First ☐

Milupa Aptamil Extra ☐

Farley's First ☐ **Go to Q10b**

Farley's Second ☐

Boots Formula 1 ☐

Boots Formula 2 ☐

Sainsburys First Menu Stage 1 milk ☐

Sainsburys First Menu Stage 2 milk ☐

Hipp Organic Infant Milk ☐

Soya-based Formula ☐
(Please cross and write in the name)

Liquid cow's milk ☐ ⇨ **Go to Q10a**

Another kind of milk ☐ ⇨ **Go to Q10b**
(Please cross and write in the name)

6

Q8. How old was your baby when you last breast fed him/her?
Please write the age in appropriate box

Either in days ☐ days

OR

In whole weeks plus any additional days ☐ weeks and ☐ days

Office Use Only

(a) What were your reasons for stopping breast feeding?
Please write in the reasons

Q9. Would you have liked to continue breast feeding for longer or had you breastfed for as long as you intended?

Would have liked to breastfeed longer ☐

I had breastfed for as long as intended ☐

5

235

Q10(a). If you use liquid cow's milk, is it whole milk, semi-skimmed or skimmed?

Whole ☐
Semi-skimmed ☐ **Go to Q11**
Skimmed ☐

(b). Thinking of the milk that you give your baby most of the time, do you normally use powdered milk, ready to feed milk or both?

Powdered ☐
Ready to feed ☐
Both ☐

Q11. Do you ever add anything to the baby milk in the bottle?

Yes ☐ ⇨ **Go to (a)**
No ☐ ⇨ **Go to Q12**

(a). What do you add to the baby milk?

Please cross one or more boxes

Sugar ☐
Honey ☐
Tea ☐
Something else *(Please cross and write in)* ☐

Q12. Where do you usually get the baby milk for your baby?

Please cross one or more boxes

From a child health clinic/hospital ☐
From a chemist shop ☐
From a supermarket ☐
From another type of shop ☐
Somewhere else *(Please cross and write in)* ☐

7

Q13. Have you always used the baby milk mentioned at Q10 or have you changed type of milk at all (apart from changing from breast milk)?

Have always used the same type of milk ☐ ⇨ **Go to Q15**
Have used other types of milk ☐ ⇨ **Go to Q14**

Q14. Why did you change types of baby milk?

Please cross one or more boxes

Baby was not satisfied/still hungry ☐
Baby kept being sick ☐
Baby was constipated ☐
Baby was allergic to the milk ☐
I preferred a different type to the one that I was given in hospital ☐
Other reason *(Please cross and write in)* ☐

Q15. Since the birth, have you received any free or reduced price milk for either yourself or your baby?

Please cross one or more boxes

Yes, baby milk for baby ☐ **Go to a)**
Yes, cows milk for myself ☐ **Go to a)**
No, neither ☐ ⇨ **Go to Q16**

(a). Where have you exchanged the tokens for milk?

Please cross one or more boxes

At the health clinic/hospital ☐
With the milkman ☐
At a supermarket ☐
At another type of shop ☐
Somewhere else *(Please cross and write in)* ☐

8

Section 3: About other drinks and food that you may give to your baby

Q16. Do you give your baby tap or mineral water to drink at the moment (including boiled tap water)?

Yes ☐
No ☐

(a) Apart from tap or mineral water, are you giving your baby anything else to drink at the moment (such as fruit juice, squash or herbal drink)?

Yes ☐ ⇨ Go to (b)
No ☐ ⇨ Go to Q18

(b) Please list the drinks giving the brand name (or say if homemade) and the flavour and say if it is a special baby drink or not.

Brand (or homemade)	Flavour	Please cross if it is a baby drink ☺

Office Use Only

Q17. Do you give your baby drinks mainly...?

Please cross one or more boxes

Because he/she is thirsty ☐
To give him/her extra vitamins ☐
To help his/her colic/wind ☐
To help his/her constipation ☐
To settle him/her ☐
Some other reason (Please cross and write in) ☐

9

Q18. Has your baby ever had any foods such as cereal, rusk or any other kind of solid food?

Yes ☐ ⇨ Go to (a)
No ☐ ⇨ Go to Q21

(a). How old was your baby when he/she first had any food apart from milk?
Please write a number in the box

Please write in the age to the nearest whole week ☐ Weeks old

Q19. At present, are you regularly giving your baby cereal, rusks or any other solid food?

Yes ☐ ⇨ Go to Q20
No ☐ ⇨ Go to Q21

Q20. Can you list all the cereal, rusks or solid food that your baby ate yesterday. Please describe each fully, giving the brand name and the stage (1 or 2) if relevant.

Didn't have solids yesterday ☐ ⇨ Go to Q21

Type of food (and stage)	Brand (or homemade)

Office Use Only

10

Section 4: *About vitamins for your baby and yourself*

Q21. Do you give your baby any extra vitamins (apart from fruit drinks mentioned at Q16)?

Yes ☐ ⇨ **Go to (a) and (b)**
No ☐ ⇨ **Go to Q22**

(a). Do you use **Children's Vitamin Drops** from the child health clinic or another brand?

Please cross one box only

Children's Vitamin Drops ☐
Other brand (*Please cross and write in*) ☐

_____

(b). How do you usually get the vitamins?

Please cross one box only

Buy the vitamins myself at the child health clinic/hospital ☐
Buy the vitamins somewhere else ☐
Get the vitamins **free** at the child clinic/hospital ☐
Get vitamins **on prescription** ☐
Other (*Please cross and describe*) ☐

_____

11

Q22. Are you taking any extra vitamin or iron supplements yourself either in tablet or powder form?

Yes ☐ ⇨ **Go to (a) and (b)**
No ☐ ⇨ **Go to Q23**

(a). What type of supplements are you taking?

Please cross one box only

Iron only ☐
Vitamins only ☐
Vitamins and iron combined ☐
Something else (*Please cross and describe*) ☐

(b). How do you usually get the vitamins or iron supplements?

Please cross one box only

Buy the vitamins or iron supplement myself at the child health clinic/hospital ☐
Buy the vitamins or iron supplements somewhere else ☐
Get the vitamins or iron supplements **free** at the child clinic/hospital ☐
Get vitamin or iron supplements **on prescription** ☐
Other (*Please cross and describe*) ☐

_____

12

Q25. Thinking back to before you had your baby, how did you plan to feed him/her?

Bottle feed ☐

Breast feed ☐ ⇨ **Go to (a)**

Breast and bottle feed ☐

Had not decided ☐ ⇨ **Go to Q26**

(a). Why did you think you would feed your baby by that method?
(Please give all your reasons and explain)

Office Use Only

14

Section 5: About *when you were pregnant*

Q23. Thinking back to when you became pregnant, did you know that increasing your intake of folic acid can be good for you in the early stages of pregnancy?

Yes ☐ ⇨ **Go to (a)**

No ☐ ⇨ **Go to Q24**

(a). Did you change your diet or take supplements to increase your intake of folic acid in the first few months of your pregnancy?

Please cross one or more boxes

Yes, I changed my diet ☐

Yes, I took supplements ☐

No neither ☐

Q24. When you were pregnant, did you take any extra vitamin or iron supplements either in tablet or powder form?

Yes ☐ ⇨ **Go to (a)**

No ☐ ⇨ **Go to Q25**

(a). What type of supplements did you take?

Please cross one or more boxes

Iron only ☐

Vitamins only ☐

Vitamins and iron combined ☐

Something else (*Please cross and describe*) ☐

13

Q26. While you were pregnant did you have any antenatal check ups?

Yes ☐ ⇒ Go to (a) and (b)
No ☐ ⇒ Go to Q27

(a). When you went for your checkups did anyone ask how you <u>planned</u> to feed your baby?

Yes ☐
No ☐

(b). At the checkups did anyone <u>discuss</u> feeding your baby with you?

Yes ☐ ⇒ Go to (c)
No ☐ ⇒ Go to Q27

(c). Who discussed feeding your baby with you?

Please cross one or more boxes

Doctor ☐
Health visitor ☐
Midwife ☐
Nurse ☐
Someone else (*Please cross and write in*) ☐
_____

15

Q27. While you were pregnant with this baby, did you go to any classes to prepare you for having the baby?

Yes ☐ ⇒ Go to (a), (b) and (c)
No ☐ ⇒ Go to Q28

(a). Who were the classes organised by?

Please cross one or more boxes

A hospital ☐
A clinic/doctor's surgery/health centre ☐
Voluntary organisation (such as the National Childbirth Trust) ☐
Someone else (*Please cross and write in*) ☐

(b). Did you attend any classes that included talks or discussions about feeding babies?

Yes ☐ ⇒ Go to (c)
No ☐ ⇒ Go to Q28

(c). Were you taught how to make up bottles of milk at the classes you attended?

Yes ☐
No ☐

Q28. While you were pregnant with this baby, did you receive advice about breastfeeding from any of the following medical staff or organisations?

Please cross one or more boxes

Doctor/GP ☐
Health visitor ☐
Midwife (including at antenatal classes) ☐ Go to Q29
Nurse (including at antenatal classes) ☐
Voluntary organisation (such as the National Childbirth Trust) ☐
Someone else (*Please cross and write in*) ☐
_____

I didn't receive any advice ☐ ⇒ Go to Q30

If you have crossed more than one box at Q28 please answer Q29.
If you have crossed only one box go to Q30

16

240

Q29. Thinking of the medical staff or organisations who gave you advice about breast feeding, who do you think gave you the most helpful advice.

Please cross one or more boxes

Doctor/GP ☐
Health visitor ☐
Midwife (including at antenatal classes) ☐
Nurse (including at antenatal classes) ☐
Voluntary organisation (such as the National Childbirth Trust) ☐
Someone else (*Please cross and write in*) ☐

_____

Q30. When you were pregnant did anyone give you any advice or information about smoking during pregnancy?

Yes ☐ ⇨ **Go to (a)**
No ☐ ⇨ **Go to Q31**

(a). Who gave you this advice?

Please cross one or more boxes

Doctor/GP ☐
Health visitor ☐
Midwife (including at antenatal classes) ☐
Nurse (including at antenatal classes) ☐
Voluntary organisation (such as the National Childbirth Trust) ☐
Friend or relative ☐
Books/leaflets/magazines ☐
Television /radio ☐
Someone else (*Please cross and write in*) ☐

_____

17

Q31. When you were pregnant did anyone give you advice or information about drinking alcohol during pregnancy?

Yes ☐ ⇨ **Go to (a)**
No ☐ ⇨ **Go to Q32**

(a). Who gave you this advice?

Please cross one or more boxes

Doctor/GP ☐
Health visitor ☐
Midwife (including at antenatal classes) ☐
Nurse (including at antenatal classes) ☐
Voluntary organisation (such as the National Childbirth Trust) ☐
Friend or relative ☐
Books/leaflets/magazines ☐
Television /radio ☐
Someone else (*Please cross and write in*) ☐

_____

Q32. Did a midwife or health visitor see you at home in connection with your pregnancy before you had the baby?

Yes, midwife ☐
Yes, health visitor ☐
No, neither ☐

Q33. Do you know any mothers with young babies?

Yes ☐ ⇨ **Go to (a)**
No ☐ ⇨ **Go to Q34**

(a). Would you say that most of the mothers you know with young babies bottle fed or breast fed?

Please cross one or more boxes

Most of them bottle fed ☐
Most of them breast fed ☐
About half of them bottle fed and half of them breast fed ☐
Don't know ☐

18

241

Q34. Do you know whether you were breast fed or bottle fed when you were a baby?

Please cross one box only

- ☐ Breast fed entirely
- ☐ Bottle fed entirely
- ☐ Both breast and bottle fed
- ☐ Don't know

Section 6: About the birth of your baby

Q35. Was your baby born in hospital or at home?

- ☐ In hospital ⇒ **Go to (a)**
- ☐ At home ⇒ **Go to Q36**

(a). How long after the baby was born did you stay in hospital?
Please enter number in one box only

Either

How many **hours** did you spend in hospital ☐ hours

Or

How many **days** did you spend in hospital ☐ days

Q36. Thinking now of the birth itself, what type of delivery did you have?

- ☐ Normal
- ☐ Forceps
- ☐ Vacuum extraction (ventouse)
- ☐ Caesarean

19

Q37. While you were in labour were you given any of these?
Please cross one or more boxes

- ☐ An epidural (spinal) injection
- ☐ Another type of injection to lessen the pain (eg pethidine)
- ☐ Gas and oxygen to breathe
- ☐ A general anaesthetic (to make you unconscious)
- ☐ Something else (*Please cross and write in*)

_____

- ☐ Nothing at all

Q38. How much did your baby weigh when he/she was born?

Either

What your baby weighed in **pounds and ounces**

☐ lbs and ☐ ozs

Or

What your baby weighed in **grams**

☐ gms

Q39. About how long after your baby was born did you first hold him/her?
Please cross one box only

- ☐ Immediately/within a few minutes
- ☐ Within an hour
- ☐ More than 1 hour, up to 12 hours
- ☐ More than 12 hours later

Q40. After the birth were you alright or was anything the matter with you?

- ☐ Alright ⇒ **Go to Q41**
- ☐ Something the matter ⇒ **Go to (a)**

(a). Did this problem affect your ability to feed your baby the way you wanted to?

- ☐ Yes
- ☐ No

20

Q41. Was your baby put into special care at all, or put under a lamp for jaundice?

Please cross one or more boxes

Yes, put into special care ☐   **Go to (a) and (b)**
Yes, put under a lamp ☐
No, neither ☐ ⇨ **Go to Q42**

(a). For how long was your baby put into special care or put under a lamp?

One day or less ☐
Two or three days ☐
Four days or more ☐

(b). Did having your baby in special care or under a lamp affect your ability to feed your baby the way you wanted to?

Yes ☐
No ☐

Q42. During the first one or two feeds, did anyone instruct you on how to put your baby to the breast yourself?

Yes ☐ ⇨ **Go to (a), (b) and (c)**
No ☐ ⇨ **Go to (c)**

(a). Who was this?

Please cross one or more boxes

Midwife ☐
Nurse ☐
Doctor ☐   **Go to (b)**
Friend/relative ☐
Someone else ☐
(Please cross and write in)

(b). Did you find this helpful?

Yes ☐   **Go to Q43**
No ☐

(c). Would you have liked any help or advice on how to put your baby to the breast?

Yes ☐
No ☐

21

Section 7: About the times that you feed your baby

If you ever breast fed your baby please answer Question 43
If your baby was completely bottle fed from birth go on to Question 45

Q43. How soon after your baby was born did you first put him/her to the breast?

Please cross one box only

Immediately/within a few minutes ☐
Within half an hour ☐
More than ° hour, up to 1 hour later ☐
More than 1 hour, up to 4 hours later ☐
More than 4 hours, up to 8 hours later ☐
More than 8 hours, up to 12 hours later ☐
More than 12 hours, up to 24 hours later ☐
More than 24 hours later ☐

If your baby was born in hospital please answer Question 44
If your baby was born at home please go on to Question 53

Q44. While you were in hospital did your baby have milk from a bottle (apart from expressed breast milk) as well as being breast fed?

Yes ☐ ⇨ **Go to (a)**
No ☐   **Go to Q47**
Don't know ☐

(a). How often did your baby have a bottle in hospital (while you were breast feeding as well)?

Please cross one box only

Once or twice only ☐
At every feed ☐
Just during the night ☐
Some other arrangements ☐   **Go to Q46**
(Please cross and describe)

Don't know ☐

22

Q48. Were there any problems feeding your baby while you were in hospital?

Yes □ ⇒ **Go to (a)**
No □ ⇒ **Go to Q50**

(a). What problems were there?
(Please describe)

Q49. Did anyone give you any help or advice about this/these problems?

Yes □ ⇒ **Go to (a)**
No □ **Go to Q50**

(a). Who helped or advised you?

Please cross one or more boxes

Midwife □
Nurse □
Doctor □
Friend / relative □
Someone else *(Please cross and write in)* □

Q50. While you were in hospital were you always able to get help or advice when you needed it?

Yes - always □
Yes - generally □
No □

Q51. When you left hospital, were you . . .

breast feeding completely □
bottle feeding completely □
or giving both breast and bottle? □

24

If your baby was completely bottle fed from birth please answer Q45 and Q46

Q45. How soon after he/she was born did you first feed your baby?

Please cross one box only

Immediately/within a few minutes □
Within half an hour □
More than ½ hour, up to 1 hour later □
More than 1 hour, up to 4 hours later □
More than 4 hours, up to 8 hours later □
More than 8 hours, up to 12 hours later □
More than 12 hours, up to 24 hours later □
More than 24 hours later □

Q46. When your baby was given a bottle of milk in hospital were you given a choice of what brand of milk you wanted to use (such as Cow and Gate, Milupa, SMA, etc)?

Yes □
No □

Section 8: About when you were in hospital

If your baby was born at home please go to Question 53

Q47. Did your baby stay beside you all the time you were in hospital?

Yes □ ⇒ **Go to Q48**
No □ ⇒ **Go to (a)**

(a). Even though he/she was not always beside you, did you always feed your baby yourself or did the midwives or nurses ever feed him/her?

Always fed baby myself □ ⇒ **Go to Q48**
Midwives/nurses sometimes fed baby □ ⇒ **Go to (b)**

(b). What did the midwives/nurses give your baby?

Please cross one or more boxes

Expressed breast milk □
Manufactured baby milk □
Dextrose or glucose water □
Water □
Don't know □

23

Q52. After you left hospital did a midwife come to visit you?

Yes □ ⇨ **Go to (a)**
No □ ⇨ **Go to Q53**

(a). How soon after you left hospital did she come?

Same day □
Next day □
Two or more days later □

Section 9: About help for you at home

Q53. After you left hospital, did you feel you knew how to get help with feeding your baby if your needed to?
(If your baby was born at home, please base your answer from when your baby was born).

Yes □
No □

Q54. Since your baby was born has a health visitor been to see you?

Yes □ ⇨ **Go to (a)**
No □ ⇨ **Go to Q55**

(a). How old was your baby when the health visitor first came?

Please write in the total number of days [ ] days old

Q55. Has your baby had a development check-up yet?

Yes □ ⇨ **Go to (a)**
No □ ⇨ **Go to Q56**

(a). Where did your baby have the development check-up?
Please cross one box only

At the child health clinic/hospital □
At your family doctor's (GP) □
At home □
Somewhere else *(Please cross and write in)* □

25

Q56. Have you received help or advice from a voluntary organisation which helps new mothers (such as the National Childbirth Trust)?

Yes □
No □

Q57. Since you left hospital have you had any problems with feeding your baby?
(If your baby was born at home, please answer about any feeding problems since the birth).

Yes □ ⇨ **Go to (a)**
No □ ⇨ **Go to Q59**

(a). What problems were there?
(Please describe)

Q58. Did anyone give you any help or advice about this/these problems?

Yes □ ⇨ **Go to (a)**
No □ ⇨ **Go to Q59**

(a). Who helped or advised you?

Please cross one or more boxes

Doctor/GP □
Health visitor □
Midwife □
Nurse □
Friend or relative □
Books/leaflets/magazines □
Someone else *(Please cross and write in)* □

Office Use Only

26

245

Q59. During your pregnancy or since the birth of your baby were you given a copy of any of these books?

Please cross one or more boxes

The Pregnancy Book ☐

The Birth to Five book ☐

"Ready Steady Baby" (Scotland only) ☐

"Breast feeding and returning to work" (Scotland only) ☐

"Breast feeding-getting off to a good start" (Scotland only) ☐

Q60. In which position do you usually place your baby to sleep?

On his/her back ☐

On his/her front ☐

On his/her side ☐

Varies ☐

Section 10: About yourself

Q61. Have you ever smoked cigarettes?

Yes ☐ ⇨ Go to (a)

No ☐ ⇨ Go to Q65

(a). Have you smoked at all in the last two years, that is since October 1998?

Yes ☐ ⇨ Go to (b)

No ☐ ⇨ Go to Q65

(b). Do you smoke cigarettes at all now?

Yes ☐ ⇨ Go to Q62

No ☐ ⇨ Go to Q63

Q62. Did you smoke cigarettes at all during pregnancy, after you found out you were pregnant?

Yes ☐ ⇨ Go to Q64

No ☐ ⇨ Go to Q65

27

Q63. When did you finally give up?

Before you knew you were pregnant ☐ **Go to Q65**

As soon as you found out you were pregnant ☐

Later on during your pregnancy ☐ **Go to Q64**

After the birth ☐

Q64. Since you knew about your pregnancy, did you do either of the following <u>during your pregnancy</u>?

Please cross one or more boxes

Cut down ☐

Gave up but started again ☐

Increased the amount you smoked ☐

None of the above ☐

Q65. During your pregnancy, did any of the people you lived with smoke cigarettes?

Yes, my partner smoked ☐

Yes, someone else I lived with smoked ☐

No, nobody else who I lived with smoked ☐

Not applicable - I lived alone ☐

(a). Do any of the people who live with you now smoke cigarettes?

Yes, my partner smokes ☐

Yes, someone else I live with smokes ☐

No, nobody else who I live with smokes ☐

Not applicable - I live alone with my baby ☐

Q66. Do you ever drink alcohol nowadays, including drinks you brew or make at home? (Please exclude low or non alcoholic drinks)

Yes ☐ ⇨ **Go to Q68**

No ☐ ⇨ **Go to Q67**

Q67. Have you drunk alcohol at all during the past two years?

Yes ☐ ⇨ **Go to Q68**

No ☐ ⇨ **Go to Q72**

28

Q68. Thinking back to when you were pregnant please cross the box that best describes how often you usually drank each of the alcoholic drinks listed below.

(Please exclude low or non alcoholic drinks)

During pregnancy I usually drank:

	Most days	3-4 times a week	Once or twice a week	Once or twice a month	Very occasionally	Not at all
Shandy	☐	☐	☐	☐	☐	☐
Beer/lager/stout/cider	☐	☐	☐	☐	☐	☐
Wine/babycham/champagne	☐	☐	☐	☐	☐	☐
Sherry/martini/vermouth/port	☐	☐	☐	☐	☐	☐
Spirits/liqueurs (eg. gin, whisky, rum, brandy, vodka)	☐	☐	☐	☐	☐	☐
Alcopops (eg. alcoholic lemonade, alcoholic colas, alcoholic fruit flavoured drinks)	☐	☐	☐	☐	☐	☐

Please check that there is a cross in one box on each line

Q69. For each type of drink you say that you had when you were pregnant, please write in the boxes the amount you usually drank each time that you had a drink.
(If none write 0)

Shandy	☐ half pints
Beer/lager/stout/cider	☐ half pints ☐ large cans ☐ small cans
Wine/babycham/champagne	☐ glasses
Sherry/martini/vermouth/port	☐ glasses
Spirits/liqueurs (eg. gin, whisky, rum, brandy, vodka)	☐ single measures (count double measures as 2)
Alcopops (e.g. alcoholic lemonade, alcoholic colas etc)	☐ bottles

29

Q70. Thinking about ALL kinds of alcoholic drinks, how often did you have an alcoholic drink of any kind during pregnancy?

Most days	☐
3-4 times a week	☐
Once or twice a week	☐
Once or twice a month	☐
Less than once a month	☐
Not at all	☐

Q71. During your pregnancy would you say you drank more, less or about the same amount of alcohol than before you were pregnant?

I drank **much more** during pregnancy than before	☐	**Go to (a)**
I drank **more** during pregnancy than before	☐	
I drank **about the same** during pregnancy as before	☐	⇨ **Go to Q72**
I drank **less** during pregnancy than before	☐	**Go to (a)**
I drank **much less** during pregnancy than before	☐	

(a). Why did you change your drinking habits during pregnancy?

Please cross one or more boxes

Drinking alcohol made me feel sick	☐
I dislike the taste of alcohol when I was pregnant	☐
Alcohol cheered me up and made me feel better	☐
Alcohol might harm my baby	☐
I had personal/family problems	☐
Some other reason *(Please cross and write in)*	☐

_____

30

Right page (Q73–Q75)

Q73. Whichever method you used to feed your baby this time, did you ever feel pushed into making this decision?

Yes, felt pushed into breastfeeding □ **Go to (a)**
Yes, felt pushed into bottlefeeding □ **Go to (a)**
No, neither □ ⇨ **Go to Q74**

(a). Who made you feel this way?

Please cross one or more boxes

Midwife □
Health visitor □
Doctor/GP □
Nurse □
Partner □
Mother □
Grandmother □
Friends/other mothers □
Voluntary organisation (eg. National Childbirth Trust) □

If your baby was entirely bottle fed from birth please go to Q76
If you ever breast fed your baby, please answer Q74

Q74. If you had another baby would you breast feed again?

Yes □
No □

If you are now completely bottle feeding your baby, go to Q76
If you are breast feeding your baby, answer Q75

Q75. For how long do you think you will continue breast feeding your baby?

Until my baby is:

Please write numbers in the boxes

Either [ ] weeks old

OR [ ] months and [ ] weeks old

Don't know/have not decided *(please cross if appropriate)* □

32

Left page (Q72)

If this is your first baby, please go on to Q73

Q72. If this is not your first baby, we would like to know how you fed your previous children. Please fill in the details below, but *do not include your latest baby.*

Previous children	Was he/she breast fed at all	If breast fed, how long did you continue breast feedings?
First child	Yes □ No □	[ ] days OR [ ] weeks OR [ ] months
Second child	Yes □ No □	[ ] days OR [ ] weeks OR [ ] months
Third child	Yes □ No □	[ ] days OR [ ] weeks OR [ ] months
Fourth child	Yes □ No □	[ ] days OR [ ] weeks OR [ ] months
Fifth child	Yes □ No □	[ ] days OR [ ] weeks OR [ ] months
Sixth child	Yes □ No □	[ ] days OR [ ] weeks OR [ ] months

31

And finally, a few questions about yourself

Q78. **What is your present age?**

Under 20 ☐
20, up to 24 ☐
25, up to 29 ☐
30, up to 34 ☐
35 or over ☐

Q79. **How old were you when you finished full-time education?** (School or college, whichever you last attended full-time)

16 or under ☐
17 ☐
18 ☐
19 or over ☐

Q80. **Are you doing any paid work at the moment?**

Yes ☐ **Go to Q81**
On paid maternity leave ☐
On unpaid maternity leave ☐
No ☐ ⇨ **Go to (a)**

(a). **Do you plan to start work again within the next two years?**

Yes, full-time ☐ **Go to Q82**
Yes, part-time ☐
No ☐
Don't know ☐

34

Q76. **Are you aware of the health benefits in breast feeding?**

Yes ☐ ⇨ **Go to (a)**
No ☐ ⇨ **Go to Q77**

(a). **What health benefits are you aware of?**
(Please describe)

The following question is about your family planning

Q77. **Since your baby was born have you used either the combined pill or mini-pill (progesterone only) to prevent pregnancy?**

Yes ☐ ⇨ **Go to (a)**
No ☐ ⇨ **Go to Q78**

(a). **How old was your baby when you began to take the pill?**

Write in how many whole weeks [ ] weeks
plus any additional days and [ ] days

33

Q82. **What was your job before you had your first baby?**
(If unemployed please describe your previous job)

Same as present job ☐ **Go to Q83**
Never worked before first baby ☐

Office Use Only
SOC
ES

(a). **What was the title of your job?**
(if you had more than one job, please give details of your main job)

(b). **What did you mainly do in your job?**
Please write in

(c). **What did the firm or organisation you worked for make or do at the site where you worked?**

(d). **Were you ...**
an employee ☐ ⇨ **Go to (e)**
or self-employed? ☐ ⇨ **Go to Q83**

(e). **Did you have any managerial duties or did you supervise any other employees?**
Yes, manager ☐
Yes, supervisor ☐
No, neither ☐

36

Q81. **What is the title of your job?**
(If you have more than one job please give details of your main job)

Office Use Only
SOC
ES

(a). **What do you mainly do in your job?**
Please write in

(b). **What does the firm or organisation you work for make or do at the site where you work?**

(c). **Are you ...**
an employee ☐ ⇨ **Go to (d)**
or self-employed? ☐ ⇨ **Go to (e)**

(d). **Do you have any managerial duties or do you supervise any other employees?**
Yes, manager ☐
Yes, supervisor ☐
No, neither ☐

(e). **Do you work mainly at home or do you go out to work?**
Mainly at home ☐
Go out to work ☐

35

Q86. **What is your ethnic group?**

Please cross one box only

White

British ☐
Irish ☐
Any other White background ☐
(please cross and write in)

Mixed

White and Black Caribbean ☐
White and Black African ☐
White and Asian ☐
Any other mixed background ☐
(please cross and write in)

Asian or Asian British

Indian ☐
Pakistani ☐
Bangladeshi ☐
Any other Asian background ☐
(please cross and write in)

Black or Black British

Caribbean ☐
African ☐
Any other Black background ☐
(please cross and write in)

Chinese or Other ethnic group

Chinese ☐
Any other ☐
(please cross and write in)

38

Q83. **Are you . . .**

married ☐ **Go to Q84**
living together ☐
single ☐ **Go to Q86**
widowed, divorced or separated? ☐

Q84. **Is your husband/partner in paid job at present?**

Yes ☐ **Go to Q85**
No ☐

Q85. **What is the title of your husband's/partner's job?**
(If unemployed, please describe his previous job)
(If he has more than one job, please give details of his main job)

Husband/partner never
had a paid job ☐ ⇨ **Go to Q86**

(a). **What does he mainly do in his job?**
Please write in

(b). **What does the firm or organisation he work for make or do at the site where he works?**

(c). **Is he . . .**

an employee ☐ ⇨ **Go to (d)**
or self-employed? ☐ ⇨ **Go to Q86**

(d). **Does he have any managerial duties or does he supervise any other employees?**

Yes, manager ☐
Yes, supervisor ☐
No, neither ☐

37

251

Q87. Is there anything else you would like to say about feeding your baby?

Yes ☐ ⇨ **Please write in below**

No ☐

Please give the date when you filled in this questionnaire

day ☐   month ☐   year ☐

Was there anything you intended to go back and complete?
Please check.

Thank you very much for your help.

We hope to contact mothers again later to see how they are feeding their babies when they are older. If the address on the envelope was not complete or if you expect to move house in the near future and know your new address, it would help us if you could write it below:

39

1154-598 England/Wales/Scotland
Stage 2

BMRB *INTERNATIONAL*

Survey of Infant Feeding

January/February 2001

E

IN CONFIDENCE

[box]

What is the questionnaire about?

This questionnaire asks about you and your new baby.

If, rather than a single baby, you have twins or triplets, please answer the questionnaire in relation to the one who was born first.

If, for any reason, your baby is no longer with you, please cross the box below and return the questionnaire to us so we do not trouble you further.

My baby is no longer with me [box]

Our guarantee of confidentiality

The names and addresses of people who co-operate in surveys are held in strict confidence by BMRB. We will never pass your name or address to any Government Department, business, the media or members of the public.

How to fill in the questionnaire

1. Most questions on the following pages can be answered simply by putting a cross in the box next to the answer that applies to you.

   Example: Yes ☒
   No ☐

   Sometimes you are asked to write in a number or the answer in your own words. Please enter numbers as figures rather than words.

2. Occasionally you may have more than one answer to a question. Please cross all the boxes next to the answers that apply to you if the instruction "**Please cross one or more boxes**" is printed on top of the boxes.

   1

3. Sometimes you are asked to give an age or a length of time in weeks and days, or days and hours. Please follow the instructions very carefully.

   For example:

   How old is your baby?

   If your baby is 15 weeks and 2 days old enter the number of whole weeks plus any additional days

   Please enter numbers in both boxes

   15 and 2
   weeks days

4. Usually after answering each question you go on to the next one unless a box you have crossed has an arrow next to it with an instruction to go to another question.

   Example: Yes ☒ ⇨ **Go to Q8.**
   No ☐

   By following the arrows carefully you will miss out some questions which do not apply, so the amount you have to fill in will make the questionnaire shorter than it looks.

5. If you cannot remember, do not know, or are unable to answer a particular question please write that in.

6. When you have finished please post the questionnaire to us as soon as possible in the reply-paid envelope provided, even if you were not able to answer all of it.

   We are very grateful for your help

   2

Section 1: About the milk that you give your baby

If you have twins or triplets please complete this questionnaire with respect to the one who was born first.

Q1. May I just check, what is your baby's first name?
Please write in below - 1 letter per box.

[ ][ ][ ][ ][ ][ ][ ][ ][ ][ ][ ]

Q2. How old is your baby?

Please write numbers in both boxes

Write in how many whole weeks plus any additional days

[ ] weeks and [ ] days

Q3. Are you still breast feeding your baby at all?

Yes [ ] ⇧ **Go to (a), (b) and (c)**
No [ ] ⇧ **Go to Q4**

(a). Do you breast feed you baby on demand or do you generally keep to set feeding times?

On demand [ ]
Generally keep to set times [ ]
It depends on the circumstances [ ]

(b). How often do you breast feed your baby now?

Once a day [ ]
Twice a day [ ]
3-4 times a day [ ]
5-6 times a day [ ]
7-8 times a day [ ]
more than 8 times a day [ ] – – – [ ]

(Please cross and write in number of times)

(c). Do you give your baby milk from a bottle at present (apart from expressed breast milk)?

Yes [ ] ⇧ **Go to Q6**
No [ ] ⇧ **Go to Q10**

Q4. How old was your baby when you last breast fed him/her?

Please write numbers in both boxes

In whole weeks plus any additional days ▢ weeks and ▢ days

(a). What were your reasons for stopping breast feeding?
Please write in the reasons

Q5. Would you have liked to continue breast feeding for longer or had you breast-fed for as long as you intended?

Would have liked to breastfeed longer ▢
I had breast fed for as long as intended ▢

5

Q6. Which kind of milk do you give your baby most of the time at the moment?

*Please cross
one box only*

Cow and Gate Premium ▢
Cow and Gate Plus ▢
Cow and Gate Omneo Comfort 1 ▢
Cow and Gate Step 1 ▢
Cow and Gate Omneo Comfort 2 ▢
Cow and Gate Next Steps ▢
SMA Gold ▢
SMA White ▢
SMA Progress ▢
Milupa Milumil ▢
Milupa Aptamil First ▢
Milupa Aptamil Extra ▢
Milupa Forward ▢
Farley's First ▢
Farley's Second ▢ ⇧ **Go to Q6b**
Farley's Follow-on milk ▢
Boots Formula 1 ▢
Boots Formula 2 ▢
Boots Follow-on milk ▢
Boots Follow-on Banana Flavour ▢
Boots Follow-on Strawberry Flavour ▢
Sainsburys First Menu Stage 1 milk ▢
Sainsburys First Menu Stage 2 milk ▢
Sainsburys First Menu Follow-on milk ▢
Hipp Organic Infant Milk ▢
Hipp Organic Follow-on Milk Drink ▢
Soya-based Formula ▢
(Please cross and write in the name)

Liquid cow's milk ▢ ⇧ **Go to Q6a**
Another kind of milk ▢ ⇧ **Go to Q6b**
(Please cross and write in the name)

6

Q6

(a). **If you use liquid cow's milk, is it whole milk, semi-skimmed or skimmed?**

Whole ☐ **Go to Q7**
Semi-skimmed ☐
Skimmed ☐

(b). **Thinking of the milk that you give your baby most of the time, do you normally use powdered milk, ready to feed milk or both?**

Powdered ☐
Ready to feed ☐
Both ☐

Q7. Do you ever add anything to the baby milk in the bottle?

Yes ☐ ⇨ **Go to (a)**
No ☐ ⇨ **Go to Q8**

(a). **What do you add to the baby milk?**

Please cross one or more boxes

Sugar ☐
Honey ☐
Tea ☐
Something else (*Please cross and write in*) ☐

_____

Q8. How old was your baby when you started giving this kind of milk?

Please write number in the box to the nearest whole week

☐☐ weeks old

7

Q9. Where do you usually get the baby milk for your baby?

Please cross one or more boxes

From a child health clinic/hospital ☐
From a chemist shop ☐
From a supermarket ☐
From another type of shop ☐
Somewhere else (*Please cross and write in*) ☐

_____

Q10. Since the time you filled in the previous questionnaire, have you received any free or reduced price milk for either yourself or your baby?

Please cross one or more boxes

Yes, baby milk for baby ☐ ⇨ **Go to a)**
Yes, cows milk for myself ☐
No, neither ☐ ⇨ **Go to Q11**

(a). **Where have you exchanged the tokens for milk?**

Please cross one or more boxes

At the health clinic/hospital ☐
With the milkman ☐
At a supermarket ☐
At another type of shop ☐
Somewhere else (*Please cross and write in*) ☐

_____

8

Q13. Do you give your baby drinks mainly...?

Please cross one or more boxes

Because he/she is thirsty ☐
To give him/her extra vitamins ☐
To help his/her colic/wind ☐
To help his/her constipation ☐
To settle him/her ☐
Some other reason
(*Please cross and write in*) ☐

_____

Q14. Has your baby ever had any foods such as cereal, rusk or any other kind of solid food?

Yes ☐ ⇨ **Go to (a).**
No ☐ ⇨ **Go to Q20**

(a). How old was your baby when he/she first had any food apart from milk?
Please write a number in the box

Please write in the age to the nearest whole week

☐ Weeks old

10

Section 2: About other drinks and food that you may give to your baby

Q11. Do you give your baby plain tap or mineral water to drink at the moment (including boiled tap water)?

Yes ☐ ⇨ **Go to a).**
No ☐ ⇨ **Go to Q12**

(a). Do you add sugar or honey to the water that you give to your baby?

Sugar ☐
Honey ☐
Neither ☐

_____

Q12. Apart from tap or mineral water, are you giving your baby anything else to drink at the moment (such as fruit juice, squash or herbal drink)?

Yes ☐ ⇨ **Go to (a).**
No ☐ ⇨ **Go to Q14**

(a). Please list the drinks giving the brand name (or say if homemade) and the flavour and say if it is a special baby drink or not.

Brand (or homemade)	Flavour	Please cross if it is a baby drink

9

257

Q15. Can you list all the cereal, rusks or solid food that your baby ate yesterday. Please describe each fully, giving the brand name or saying if it is home made. For commercial baby food, please tick the column to show whether it was dried or tinned/jarred.

Didn't have solids yesterday ☐ ⇨ **Go to Q16**

Type of food (and stage)	Brand (or homemade)	Please tick to show whether	
		Dried	Tinned/Jarred

Q16. Do you use milk to mix up your baby's food?

Yes ☐ ⇨ **Go to (a).**
No ☐ ⇨ **Go to Q17**

(a). Do you usually use

Infant formula milk ☐
or Liquid cow's milk ☐
or something else **(please cross and write in)** ☐

Q17. When you give your baby solid food, do you give him/her fruit juice or other drinks containing vitamin C at the same time?

Yes, usually ☐
Yes, sometimes ☐
No ☐

11

Q18. Does your baby usually have three meals of solid food a day?

Yes ☐ **Go to (a).**
No ☐ **Go to Q19**

(a). How old was your baby when he/she regularly started having three meals of solid foods a day?

Please write in the age to the nearest whole week

☐ Weeks old

Q19. What do you take into account when deciding what solid foods to give your baby?
Please write in

12

Section 3: About vitamins for your baby and yourself

Q20. Do you give your baby any extra vitamins (apart from fruit drinks mentioned at Q12)?

Yes ☐ ⇨ **Go to (a) and (b)**
No ☐ ⇨ **Go to Q21**

(a). Do you use Children's Vitamin Drops from the child health clinic or another brand?

*Please cross
one box only*

Children's Vitamin Drops ☐
Other brand (*Please cross and write in*) ☐

_____

(b). How do you usually get the vitamins?

*Please cross
one box only*

Buy the vitamins myself at the child
health clinic/hospital ☐
Buy the vitamins somewhere else ☐
Get the vitamins **free** at the child clinic/hospital ☐
Get vitamins **on prescription** ☐
Other (*Please cross and describe*) ☐

_____

13

Q21. Are you taking any extra vitamin or iron supplements yourself either in tablet or powder form?

Yes ☐ ⇨ **Go to (a) and (b)**
No ☐ ⇨ **Go to Q22**

(a). What type of supplements are you taking?

*Please cross
one box only*

Iron only ☐
Vitamins only ☐
Vitamins and iron combined ☐
Something else (*Please cross and describe*) ☐

(b). How do you usually get the vitamins or iron supplements?

*Please cross
one box only*

Buy the vitamins or iron supplement myself
at the child health clinic/hospital ☐
Buy the vitamins or iron supplements
somewhere else ☐
Get the vitamins or iron supplements **free** at the
child clinic/hospital ☐
Get vitamin or iron supplements **on prescription** ☐
Other (*Please cross and describe*) ☐

_____

14

Section 4: About check-ups for your baby

Q22. Do you take your baby to a child health clinic for advice or regular check-ups?

Yes, for advice or regular check-ups ☐ ⇨ **Go to (a).**

No ☐ ⇨ **Go to Q23**

(a). About how often do you take your baby to a child health clinic?

Please cross one box only

Once a week ☐

Once a fortnight ☐

Once a month ☐

Less than once a month ☐

Q23. Do you take your baby to your family doctor (GP) for advice or regular check-ups?

Yes, for advice or regular check-ups ☐ ⇨ **Go to (a).**

No ☐ ⇨ **Go to Q24**

(a). About how often do you take your baby to your family doctor (GP) for advice or regular check-ups?

Please cross one box only

Once a week ☐

Once a fortnight ☐

Once a month ☐

Less than once a month ☐

15

Section 5: About advice for you about feeding your baby

Q24. Have you had any problems with feeding your baby since the time when you filled in the previous questionnaire?

Yes ☐ ⇨ **Go to (a).**

No ☐ ⇨ **Go to Q26**

(a). **What problems have you had?** *(Please describe)*

Q25. Did anyone give you help or advice about these problems?

Yes ☐ ⇨ **Go to (a).**

No ☐

Have not asked for help or advice ☐ **Go to Q26**

(a). **Who helped or advised you?**

Please cross one or more boxes

Doctor/GP ☐

Health visitor ☐

Nurse ☐

Voluntary organisation (such as the National Childbirth Trust) ☐

Friend or Relative ☐

Books/leaflets/magazines ☐

Someone else *(please cross and write in)* ☐

_____

16

Q26. Has anyone given you help or advice on breast feeding since the time you filled in the previous questionnaire?

Yes ☐ ⇨ **Go to (a).**
No ☐ **Go to Q27**
Have not asked for help or advice ☐

(a). Who helped or advised you on breast feeding?

*Please cross one
or more boxes*

Doctor/GP ☐
Health visitor ☐
Nurse ☐
Voluntary organisation (such as the National Childbirth Trust) ☐
Friend or Relative ☐
Books/leaflets/magazines ☐
Someone else (*please cross and write in*) ☐
_____

Q27. Have you ever wanted or tried to feed your baby when you were out in public places?

Yes ☐ ⇨ **Go to (a)**
No ☐ ⇨ **Go to Q28**

(a) Have you ever had problems finding somewhere to feed your baby when you were out in public places?

Yes ☐
No ☐

17

Q28. Have you ever breast fed your baby in a public place?
(*Please exclude hospitals*)

Yes ☐ ⇨ **Go to (a).**
No ☐ **Go to Q29**
Bottle fed from birth ☐

(a). When you have breast fed in a public place do you:

*Please cross one
box only*

prefer a mother and baby room? ☐
prefer to breastfeed without going to any special place? ☐
no preference ☐

Q29. Where do you think that it is important to have facilities for feeding babies?

*Please cross one
or more boxes*

Shops/shopping centres ☐
Restaurants ☐
Public toilets ☐
Other places (*please cross and write in*) ☐
_____

Section 6: About yourself

Q30. Do you smoke cigarettes at all nowadays?

Yes ☐ ⇨ **Go to (a).**
No ☐ ⇨ **Go to Q31**

(a) About how many cigarettes a <u>day</u> do you usually smoke now?

Please write a number in the box ☐

18

Section 7: About your plans for work

Q34. Are you doing any paid work at the moment?

Yes	[ ]
On paid maternity leave	[ ] Go to Q35
On unpaid maternity leave	[ ]
No	[ ] ⇒ Go to (a).

(a). Do you intend to return to work within the next year?

Yes	[ ] ⇒ Go to Q38
No	[ ] ⇒ Go to Q40

Q35. What is the title of your job (including where you are on maternity leave)?
(If you have more than one job please give details of your main job)

(a). What do you mainly do in your job?
Please write in

(b). What does the firm or organisation you work for make or do at the site where you work?

(c). Are you …

an employee	[ ]
or self-employed?	[ ]

(d). Do you have any managerial duties or do you supervise any other employees?

Yes, manager	[ ]
Yes, supervisor	[ ]
No, neither	[ ]

(e). Do you work mainly at home or do you go out to work?

Mainly at home	[ ]
Go out to work	[ ]

[20]

Q31. Does your husband/partner smoke cigarettes at all nowadays?

Yes	[ ] ⇒ Go to (a).
No	[ ] Go to Q32
No partner	[ ]

(a) About how many cigarettes a day does your husband/partner usually smoke now?

Please write the number in the box [ ]

Q32. And do you live with anyone else (other than a husband/partner) who smokes?

Yes	[ ]
No	[ ]

The following question is about your use of contraception.

Q33. Since your baby was born have you used either the combined pill or mini-pill (progesterone only) to prevent pregnancy?

Yes	[ ] ⇒ Go to (a).
No	[ ] ⇒ Go to Q34

(a) How old was your baby when you began to take the pill?

Please write in how many weeks to the nearest whole week [ ]

[19]

If you are currently on paid or unpaid maternity leave, please answer Q37
If you are currently working, please answer Q40

Q37. Do you intend to return to work when your maternity leave has come to an end?

Yes ☐ ⇒ **Go to Q38**
No ☐ ⇒ **Go to Q40**
Undecided ☐

Q38. What age will your baby be when you return to work?

4 months, less than 5 months ☐
5 months, less than 6 months ☐
6 months, less than 9 months ☐
9 months, less than 1 year ☐
1 year or older ☐
Undecided ☐

(a). How many hours do you intend to work?

Less than 15 ☐
15, less than 30 ☐
31 or more hours ☐
Will vary ☐
Undecided ☐

(b). What type of childcare do you intend to use?
Please cross one or more boxes

Childminder/Nanny ☐
Work-place creche or nursery ☐
Other creche or nursery ☐
Husband or partner ☐
The child's grandparent(s) ☐
Another relative ☐
Friend ☐
Other person/place (*Please describe*) ☐
_____
Not yet decided ☐
Do not intend to use any childcare ☐

22

If you are currently working, please answer Q36
If you are currently on paid or unpaid maternity leave, please answer Q37

Q36. How many hours a week do you work?

Less than 15 ☐
15, less than 30 ☐
31 or more hours ☐
Varies ☐

(a). How is your baby cared for while you are at work?
Please cross one or more boxes

Childminder/Nanny ☐
Work-place creche or nursery ☐
Other creche or nursery ☐
Husband or partner ☐
The child's grandparent(s) ☐
Another relative ☐
Friend ☐
Other person/place (*Please describe*) ☐
_____
Do not use any childcare ☐

(b). Has your return to work affected the way in which you are feeding your baby at all?

Yes ☐ ⇒ **Go to c)**
No ☐ ⇒ **Go to Q40**

(c). How has this affected the way in which you feed your baby?
Please write in

Now go to Q40

21

Q39. Do you think your return to work will affect the way in which you feed your baby?

Yes ☐ Go to a).
No ☐ Go to Q40

(a). How do you think that this will affect the way in which you feed your baby?
(Please write in)

Q40. Is there anything else you would like to say about feeding your baby?

Yes ☐ ⇒ **Please write in below**
No ☐

Please give the date when you filled in this questionnaire

day   month   year

2001

23

Please turn over

Was there anything you intended to go back and complete?
Please check.

Thank you very much for your help.

We hope to contact mothers again later to see how they are feeding their babies when they are older. If the address on the envelope was not complete or if you expect to move house in the near future and know your new address, it would help us if you could write it below:

24

1154-598 England/Wales/Scotland
Stage 3

BMRB *INTERNATIONAL*

Survey of Infant Feeding
June/July 2001

IN CONFIDENCE

[ ]   G

What is the questionnaire about?

This questionnaire asks about you and your new baby.

If, rather than a single baby, you have twins or triplets, please answer the questionnaire in relation to the one who was born first.

If, for any reason, your baby is no longer with you, please cross the box below and return the questionnaire to us so we do not trouble you further.

My baby is no longer with me   [ ]

Our guarantee of confidentiality

The names and addresses of people who co-operate in surveys are held in strict confidence by BMRB International. We will never pass your name or address to any Government Department, business, the media or members of the public.

How to fill in the questionnaire

1. Most questions on the following pages can be answered simply by putting a cross in the box next to the answer that applies to you.

   Example: Yes [X]   No [ ]

   Sometimes you are asked to write in a number or the answer in your own words. Please enter numbers as figures rather than words.

2. Occasionally you may have more than one answer to a question. Please cross all the boxes next to the answers that apply to you if the instruction **"Please cross one or more boxes"** is printed on top of the boxes.

[1]

---

3. Sometimes you are asked to give an age or a length of time in weeks and days, or days and hours. Please follow the instructions very carefully.

   For example:

   How old is your baby?

   If your baby is 15 weeks and 2 days old enter the number of whole weeks plus any additional days

   Please enter numbers in both boxes

   [15] and [2]
   weeks   days

4. Usually after answering each question you go on to the next one unless a box you have crossed has an arrow next to it with an instruction to go to another question.

   Example: Yes [X] ⇒ **Go to Q8.**
           No [ ]

   By following the arrows carefully you will miss out some questions which do not apply, so the amount you have to fill in will make the questionnaire shorter than it looks.

5. If you cannot remember, do not know, or are unable to answer a particular question please write that in.

6. When you have finished please post the questionnaire to us as soon as possible in the reply-paid envelope provided, even if you were not able to answer all of it.

We are very grateful for your help

[2]

Section 1: About the milk that you give your baby

If you have twins or triplets please complete this questionnaire with respect to the one who was born first.

Q1. May I just check, what is your baby's first name?
Please write in below – 1 letter per box.

☐☐☐☐☐☐☐☐☐☐☐☐

Q2. How old is your baby?

Write in how many whole weeks plus any additional days

Please write numbers in both boxes

☐ weeks   and   ☐ days

3

Q3. Are you still breast feeding your baby at all?

Yes ☐ ⇧ Go to (a), (b) and (c)
No ☐ ⇧ Go to Q4

(a). Do you breast feed your baby on demand or do you generally keep to set feeding times?

On demand ☐
Generally keep to set times ☐
It depends on the circumstances ☐

(b). How often do you breast feed your baby now?

Once a day ☐
Twice a day ☐
3–4 times a day ☐
5–6 times a day ☐
7–8 times a day ☐
more than 8 times a day ☐
(Please cross and write in number of times) ☐

(c). Do you give your baby milk from a bottle or cup at present (apart from expressed breast milk)?

Yes ☐ ⇧ Go to Q6
No ☐ ⇧ Go to Q14

4

Q4. How old was your baby when you last breast fed him/her?

Please write numbers in both boxes

In whole weeks plus any additional days [ ] weeks and [ ] days

(a). What were your reasons for stopping breast feeding?
Please write in the reasons

Q5. Would you have liked to continue breast feeding for longer or had you breast-fed for as long as you intended?

Would have liked to have breast fed longer [ ]
I had breast fed for as long as intended [ ] Go to Q7

Q6. Do you mainly breast feed your baby at the moment or do you mainly use formula or cow's milk?

Please cross one box only

Mainly breast feed [ ]
Mainly use formula or cow's milk [ ]
Use about the same amount of both types of milk [ ]

5

Q7. Which kind of milk do you give your baby most of the time at the moment?

Please cross one box only

Cow and Gate Premium [ ]
Cow and Gate Plus [ ]
Cow and Gate Omneo Comfort 1 [ ]
Cow and Gate Step 1 [ ]
Cow and Gate Omneo Comfort 2 [ ]
Cow and Gate Next Steps [ ]
SMA Gold [ ]
SMA White [ ]
SMA Progress [ ]
Milupa Milumil [ ]
Milupa Aptamil First [ ]
Milupa Aptamil Extra [ ]
Milupa Forward [ ]
Farley's First [ ]
Farley's Second [ ] ⇨ Go to Q8
Farley's Follow-on milk [ ]
Boots Formula 1 [ ]
Boots Formula 2 [ ]
Boots Follow-on milk [ ]
Boots Follow-on Banana Flavour [ ]
Boots Follow-on Strawberry Flavour [ ]
Sainsburys First Menu Stage 1 milk [ ]
Sainsburys First Menu Stage 2 milk [ ]
Sainsburys First Menu Follow-on milk [ ]
Hipp Organic Infant Milk [ ]
Hipp Organic Follow-on Milk Drink [ ]
Soya-based Formula [ ]
(Please cross and write in the name)

Liquid cow's milk [ ] ⇨ Go to Q11
Another kind of milk [ ] ⇨ Go to Q8
(Please cross and write in the name)

6

Q8. Thinking of the milk that you give your baby most of the time, do you normally use powdered milk, ready to feed milk or both?

Powdered ☐
Ready to feed ☐
Both ☐

Q9. How old was your baby when you started giving this kind of milk?

Please write the age in the box to the nearest whole week

☐ weeks old

Q10. Do you ever give your baby liquid cow's milk at the moment?

Yes ☐ ⇨ Go to Q11
No ☐ ⇨ Go to Q13

Q11. Do you use whole, semi-skimmed or skimmed liquid cow's milk?

Please cross one or more boxes

Whole ☐
Semi-skimmed ☐
Skimmed ☐

Q12. How old was your baby when you started giving liquid cow's milk?

Please write the age in the box to the nearest whole week

☐ weeks old

7

Q13. Do you ever add anything to the baby milk in the bottle?

Yes ☐ ⇨ Go to (a)
No ☐ ⇨ Go to Q14

(a). What do you add to the milk?

Please cross one or more boxes

Sugar ☐
Honey ☐
Tea ☐

Something else *(Please cross and write in)* ☐

_____

Q14. Since the time you filled in the previous questionnaire, have you received any free or reduced price milk for either yourself or your baby?

Please cross one or more boxes

Yes, baby milk for baby ☐ Go to (a)
Yes, cows milk for myself ☐
No, neither ☐ ⇨ Go to Q15

(a). Where have you exchanged the tokens for milk?

Please cross one or more boxes

At the health clinic/hospital ☐
With the milkman ☐
At a supermarket ☐
At another type of shop ☐

Somewhere else *(Please cross and write in)* ☐

_____

8

Q15. Has your baby ever drunk from a cup or beaker with a spout?

Yes ☐ Go to (a)
No ☐ Go to Q16

(a). How old was your baby when he/she began to use the cup or beaker?

[ ] weeks old

Please write the age in the box to the nearest whole week

Q16. Does your baby use a dummy at present?

Yes ☐
No ☐

9

Section 2: About other drinks and food that you may give to your baby

Q17. Do you give your baby plain tap or mineral water to drink at the moment (including boiled tap water)?

Yes ☐ ⇒ Go to (a)
No ☐ ⇒ Go to Q18

(a). Do you add sugar or honey to the water that you give to your baby?

Sugar ☐
Honey ☐
Neither ☐

Q18. Apart from tap or mineral water, are you giving your baby anything else to drink at the moment (such as fruit juice, squash or herbal drink)?

Yes ☐ ⇒ Go to (a)
No ☐ ⇒ Go to Q19

(a). Please list the drinks giving the brand name (or say if homemade) and the flavour and say if it is a special baby drink or not.

Brand (or homemade)	Flavour	Please cross if it is a baby drink

10

The following questions are about the food that you give to your baby.

Q19. Has your baby ever had any foods such as cereal, rusk or any other kind of solid food?

Yes ☐ ⇨ Go to (a)

No ☐ ⇨ Go to Q32

(a). How old was your baby when he/she first had any food apart from milk?
Please write a number in the box

☐ Weeks old

Please write in the age to the nearest whole week

Q20. Can you list all the cereal, rusks or solid food that your baby ate yesterday. Please describe each fully, giving the brand name or saying if it is home made. For commercial baby food, please tick the column to show whether it was dried or tinned/jarred.

Didn't have solids yesterday ☐ ⇨ Go to Q21

Type of food (and stage)	Brand (or homemade)	Please tick to show whether	
		Dried	Tinned/Jarred

11

Q21. Do you ever use liquid cow's milk to mix up your baby's food?

Yes ☐ ⇨ Go to (a)

No ☐ ⇨ Go to Q22

(a). How old was your baby when you first used liquid cow's milk to mix up your baby's food?

☐ weeks old

Please write in the age to the nearest whole week

Q22. Do you use any other type of milk to mix up your baby's food?

Yes ☐ ⇨ Go to (a)

No ☐ ⇨ Go to Q23

(a). What types of milk do you usually use?

Please cross one or more boxes

Infant formula milk ☐

Follow on formula milk ☐

Expressed breast milk ☐

Something else (*Please cross and write in*) ☐

Q23. When you give your baby solid food, do you give him/her fruit juice or other drinks containing vitamin C at the same time?

Yes, usually ☐

Yes, sometimes ☐

No ☐

12

Q24. How often do you usually give your baby the following types of foods nowadays?

Please cross one box in each row

Type of food	More than once a day	Once a day	3 or more times a week	Once or twice a week	Less than once a week	Never
Cereals or Rusks	☐	☐	☐	☐	☐	☐
Rice or Pasta	☐	☐	☐	☐	☐	☐
Bread	☐	☐	☐	☐	☐	☐
Meat	☐	☐	☐	☐	☐	☐
Fish (including tuna)	☐	☐	☐	☐	☐	☐
Eggs	☐	☐	☐	☐	☐	☐
Potatoes	☐	☐	☐	☐	☐	☐
Peas, beans, lentils or chickpeas	☐	☐	☐	☐	☐	☐
Raw vegetables	☐	☐	☐	☐	☐	☐
Cooked vegetables	☐	☐	☐	☐	☐	☐
Raw fruit	☐	☐	☐	☐	☐	☐
Cooked fruit	☐	☐	☐	☐	☐	☐
Cheese, yoghurt, fromage frais	☐	☐	☐	☐	☐	☐
Puddings or desserts	☐	☐	☐	☐	☐	☐
Sweets or chocolate	☐	☐	☐	☐	☐	☐

Q25. Do you ever give your baby home made solid foods?

Yes ☐
No ☐

Q26. How would you describe the variety of foods that your baby generally eats? Does he/she...

Please cross one box only

eat most things ☐
eat a reasonable variety of things ☐
or is he/she a fussy or faddy eater ☐

13

Q27. Do you avoid giving your baby foods with particular ingredients?

Yes ☐ ⇨ Go to (a)
No ☐ ⇨ Go to Q28

(a). Which ingredients do you avoid and why?

Ingredient	Reason for avoiding

Q28. Has your baby ever been given meat or food with meat in it?

Yes ☐ ⇨ Go to (a)
No ☐ ⇨ Go to Q29

(a). How often do you give your baby meat or food with meat in it at the moment?

Please cross one box only

Every day ☐
3 or 4 times a week ☐
1 or 2 times a week ☐ Go to Q30
About once every 2 weeks ☐
Less often than once every 2 weeks ☐
I never give meat at the moment ☐ ⇨ Go to Q29

14

271

Section 3: About vitamins for your baby and yourself

Q32. Do you give your baby any extra vitamins (apart from fruit drinks mentioned at Q18)?

Yes ☐ ⇒ Go to (a) and (b)

No ☐ ⇒ Go to Q33

(a). Do you use Children's Vitamin Drops from your clinic or do you get another brand from a shop?

Children's Vitamin Drops ☐

Other brand from a shop ☐

(Please cross box and write full name below)

_____

(b). How do you usually get the vitamins?

*Please cross
one box only*

Buy the vitamins myself at my clinic ☐

Buy the vitamins from a shop ☐

Get the vitamins free at my clinic ☐

Get vitamins on prescription ☐

Other *(Please cross and describe)* ☐

_____

16

Q29. Why don't you give your baby meat or food with meat in it?

*Please cross
one box only*

My baby doesn't like meat ☐

I don't think my baby is ready for meat yet ☐

I intend to give my baby a vegetarian diet ☐

Some other reason *(Please cross and write in)* ☐

_____

Q30. Has it been difficult to wean your baby onto solid food?

Yes ☐ ⇒ Go to (a)

No ☐ ⇒ Go to Q31

(a). In what way has it been difficult?

*Please cross
one or more
boxes*

Baby would not take solids ☐

Baby would only take certain solids ☐

Baby was disinterested in food ☐

Baby prefers drinks to food ☐

Baby vomiting ☐

Some other reason *(Please cross and write in)* ☐

_____

Q31. Has your baby ever fed him/herself using a spoon?

Yes ☐ ⇒ Go to (a)

No ☐ ⇒ Go to Q32

(a). How old was your baby when he/she began to use a spoon?

Please write in the age to the nearest whole week ☐☐ weeks old

15

Q33. Are you taking any extra vitamin or iron supplements <u>yourself</u> either in tablet or powder form?

Yes ⇨ Go to (a)
No ⇨ Go to Q34

(a). What type of supplements are you taking?

Please cross one box only

Iron only ☐
Vitamins only ☐
Vitamins and iron combined ☐
Something else (*Please cross and describe*) ☐
_____

17

Section 5: About advice for you about feeding your baby

Q34. Have you had any problems with feeding your baby since the time when you filled in the previous questionnaire?

Yes ⇨ Go to (a)
No ⇨ Go to Q36

(a). What problems have you had?
(*Please describe*)

Q35. Did you get help or advice about these problems?

Yes ⇨ Go to (a)
No ☐
Did not ask for help or advice ☐ Go to Q36

(a). Who helped or advised you?

Please cross one or more boxes

Doctor/GP ☐
Health visitor ☐
Nurse ☐
Voluntary organisation (such as the National Childbirth Trust) ☐
Friend or Relative ☐
Books/leaflets/magazines ☐
TV or Radio ☐
Someone else (*please cross and write in*) ☐
_____

18

Q36. Thinking back since your baby was born, who or what has been the most helpful in giving you general advice on feeding your baby?

Please cross one or more boxes

Doctor/GP ☐
Health visitor ☐
Nurse ☐
Midwife ☐
Voluntary organisation (e.g. National Childbirth Trust) ☐
Friend or Relative ☐
Books/leaflets/magazines ☐
TV or Radio ☐
Someone else (*please cross and write in*) ☐

Section 6: About yourself

Q37. Do you smoke cigarettes at all nowadays?

Yes ☐
No ☐

The following question is about your use of contraception.

Q38. Since your baby was born have you used either the combined pill or mini-pill (progesterone only) to prevent pregnancy?

Yes - combined pill ☐ ⇨ Go to (a)
Yes - mini-pill ☐ ⇨ Go to (a)
No ☐ Go to Q39

(a) How old was your baby when you began to take the pill?

Please write in how many weeks to the nearest whole week ☐

19

Section 7: About your plans for work

Q39. Are you doing any paid work at the moment?

Yes ☐ Go to Q40
On paid maternity leave ☐
On unpaid maternity leave ☐
No ☐ ⇨ Go to (a)

(a) Do you intend to return to work within the next year?

Yes ☐ ⇨ Go to Q44
No ☐ ⇨ Go to Q46

Q40. What is the title of your job (including where you are on maternity leave)?
(*If you have more than one job please give details of your main job*)

(a) What do you mainly do in your job?
Please write in

(b) What does the firm or organisation you work for make or do at the site where you work?

(c) Are you . . .
an employee ☐
or self-employed ☐

(d) Do you have any managerial duties or do you supervise any other employees?
Yes, manager ☐
Yes, supervisor ☐
No, neither ☐

(e) Do you work mainly at home or do you go out to work?
Mainly at home ☐ ⇨ Go to Q42
Go out to work ☐ ⇨ Go to Q41

20

Q41. How is your baby usually provided with milk while you are at work?

Please cross one or more boxes

Baby is given formula milk ☐

Baby is given cow's milk ☐

I take him/her to work so that I can breast feed/ I breast feed at work-place creche ☐

I express breast milk for him/her to have while I am at work ☐

Baby has other milk while I am at work ☐

Baby does not have milk while I am at work ☐

Other arrangement (*Please cross and describe*) ☐

_____

21

If you are currently working, please answer Q42
If you are currently on paid or unpaid maternity leave, please go to Q43

Q42. How many hours a week do you work?

Less than 15 ☐

15 to 30 hours ☐

31 or more hours ☐

Varies ☐

(a). How is your baby cared for while you are at work?

Please cross one or more boxes

Childminder/Nanny ☐

Work-place creche or nursery ☐

Other creche or nursery ☐

Husband or partner ☐

The child's grandparent(s) ☐

Another relative ☐

Friend ☐

Other person/place (*Please describe*) ☐

_____

Do not use any childcare ☐

(b). Has your return to work affected the way in which you are feeding your baby at all?

Yes ☐ ⇨ Go to (c)

No ☐ ⇨ Go to Q46

(c). How has this affected the way in which you feed your baby?
Please write in

_____

Now go to Q46

22

If you are currently on paid or unpaid maternity leave, please answer Q43
If you are currently working, please go to Q46

Q43. Do you intend to return to work when your maternity leave has come to an end?

Yes ☐ ⇨ Go to Q44
No ☐ ⇨ Go to Q46
Undecided ☐

Q44. What age will your baby be when you return to work?

6 months, less than 9 months ☐
9 months, less than 1 year ☐
1 year or older ☐
Undecided ☐

(a). How many hours do you intend to work?

Less than 15 ☐
15 to 30 hours ☐
31 or more hours ☐
Will vary ☐
Undecided ☐

(b). What type of childcare do you intend to use?

Please cross one or more boxes

Childminder/Nanny ☐
Work-place creche or nursery ☐
Other creche or nursery ☐
Husband or partner ☐
The child's grandparent(s) ☐
Another relative ☐
Friend ☐
Other person/place *(Please describe)* ☐

Not yet decided ☐
Do not intend to use any childcare ☐

Q45. Do you think your return to work will affect the way in which you feed your baby?

Yes ☐ ⇨ Go to (a)
No ☐ ⇨ Go to Q46

(a). How do you think that this will affect the way in which you feed your baby?
(Please write in)

Q46. When you look back on how you have fed your baby since birth are you happy with everything you decided to do or do you wish that you had made other decisions about feeding your baby?

Happy with my decisions ⇨ Go to Q47
Wish that I had made other decisions ⇨ Go to (a)

(a). What other decisions would you have made?

Q47. Is there anything else you would like to say about feeding your baby?

Yes ☐ ⇨ **Please write in below**

No ☐

Please give the date when you filled in this questionnaire

day month year

☐ ☐ 2001

Was there anything you intended to go back and complete?
Please check.

Thank you very much for your help.

25